**LOAN PERIODS**

# Paediatric Neurosurgery

## A handbook for the multidisciplinary team

LINDY MAY

RGN, RSCN, MSc(Neuroscience), Diploma in Counselling
Great Ormond Street Hospital for Children NHS Trust, London

W

WHURR PUBLISHERS

LONDON AND PHILADELPHIA

© 2001 Whurr Publishers Ltd

First published 2001 by Whurr Publishers Ltd
19b Compton Terrace, London N1 2UN, England
325 Chestnut Street, Philadelphia PA 19106, USA

1009966645

**British Library Cataloguing in Publication Data**
A catalogue record for this book is available from the
British Library.

ISBN 1 86156 224 1

Printed and bound in the UK by Athenaeum Press Ltd,
Gateshead, Tyne & Wear

# Contents

# Preface

The growth of co-operation between disciplines when caring for the paediatric neurosurgical patient in recent years has been admirable. As demands increase, so the skills of the multidisciplinary team have adapted, progressed and developed to keep pace with the changing needs and requirements of the child. All members of the team should contribute in promoting good neuroprotection and rehabilitation for the child and should be able to assist in research-based and evidence-based practice. According to family systems theory, anything that affects one member of the family affects the whole family; therefore the multidisciplinary team must provide joint decision making and integrated family care whenever possible.

Children fortunately suffer from fewer neurosurgical illnesses than adults; this partly explains why there are few paediatric neurosurgical departments throughout the world, although cost and location are also important factors. It is therefore important that communication and education are shared across units, be this in the form of conferences, e-mail, and such working groups as the British Paediatric Neurosurgical Nursing Benchmarking Group.

The aim of the book is to pull together the main themes surrounding the paediatric neurosurgical patient; it is an abbreviated summary of a very complex subject and does not set out to cover every aspect of the needs of these children.

The first chapter gives an overview of the anatomy and physiology of the central nervous system, signs and symptoms of raised intracranial pressure, and the main neurodiagnostic procedures used in children. Chapter 2 describes the vast topic of hydrocephalus in children, subdural haematoma and the rare condition of benign intracranial hypertension (BIH). Chapter 3 describes the care of children with congenital spinal abnormalities including all forms of spina bifida and the more unusual craniovertebral abnormalities of childhood. Chapter 4 guides the reader through the vast subject of paediatric central nervous system tumours, including surgery, radiotherapy, chemotherapy and palliative care. Chapter 5 outlines the care of the child undergoing surgery for intractable epilepsy. The complex care requirements of the child following head injury are the subject of Chapter 6, and Chapter 7 describes the skull abnormalities of craniosynostosis and the associated surgical intervention and care. Chapter 8 describes congenital abnormalities of the brain, including encephalocoeles, cysts and Arnold Chiari malformations. Chapter 9 describes the main vascular abnormalities of childhood and the treatment and care required.

Each chapter ends with a section written by a parent and child. It is hoped that we will learn from their thoughts and that our care will be improved from a deeper understanding of their feelings. Many of the parents have found it cathartic to write, and have also learned more about their child's feelings.

Those interested in this group of children are, by nature, inquisitive and challenging. It is hoped that this book will provide education and interest and will stimulate further developments in this field.

# Acknowledgements

I wish to thank those health care professionals at Great Ormond Street Hospital for Children NHS Trust, London, who have advised me on the content and have diligently proofread stages of the book: Fiona Blackwell, William Harkness, Richard Hayward, Kim Phipps, Nikki Shack, Dominic Thompson.

## Dedication

This book is dedicated to all the children and families who have taught us so much. They make us humble in their ability to cope. It is dedicated to my nursing colleagues, whose enthusiasm and expertise have kept me stimulated and motivated. And finally, it is dedicated to my family, for their interest and encouragement in my work.

# Chapter 1
# Anatomy and physiology

This chapter provides an overview of essential neuroanatomy and neuro-physiology, to enable readers to refresh their knowledge and to use the book without frequent reference to other texts. It does not attempt to provide a concise or complete picture of the nervous system, as this huge field is best covered by books dedicated purely to that subject.

The nervous system is a vast communications network, divided anatomically into the central nervous system (CNS) and the peripheral nervous system (PNS). Consisting of 100 billion nerve cells, the central nervous system could be described as a telephone system of a huge city whereas the other major regulatory system of the body – the endocrine system – could be described as the postal service of that city. The CNS is situated inside the body and has to be kept in touch with both the body and the world outside it. The peripheral nerves are the 'telephone wires' that provide this connection by means of cables of nerve fibres that bring messages to and from the CNS.

The central nervous system consists of the brain and spinal cord. The peripheral nervous system is composed of the cranial and spinal bones, the somatic and visceral systems (both with efferent and afferent divisions) and the autonomic nervous system, with its sympathetic and parasympathetic divisions. This complex system of feedback mechanisms enables the brain and spinal cord to communicate with the entire body.

Outside the CNS (the peripheral nerves, connecting muscles, skin and other organ systems) the bundles of axons are called nerves. There are 31 pairs of spinal nerves and 12 pairs of cranial nerves.

The spinal nerves in the cervical spine (C1 to C7) exit over their corresponding vertebrae, the remaining nerves exiting below their corresponding vertebrae. The spinal cord is shorter than the vertebral column, ending at about L2, with nerves L3–S5 continuing as the corda equina.

Roughly speaking, the cranial nerves and their nuclei are apportioned equally between the three brain segments (CNs 1, 2, 3, 4 in the mid brain; CNs 5, 6, 7, 8 in the pons; CNs 9, 10, 11, 12 in the medulla).

1

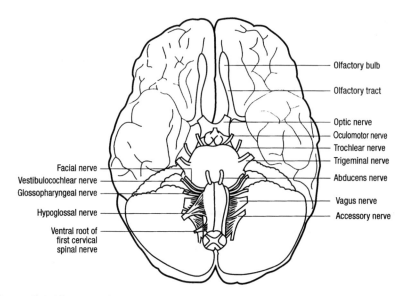

Olfactory bulb
Olfactory tract
Optic nerve
Oculomotor nerve
Trochlear nerve
Trigeminal nerve
Abducens nerve
Vagus nerve
Accessory nerve

Facial nerve
Vestibulocochlear nerve
Glossopharyngeal nerve
Hypoglossal nerve
Ventral root of
first cervical
spinal nerve

**Figure 1.1.** The cranial nerves.

The cranial nerves are as follows:

| | |
|---|---|
| CN1: | olfactory nerve (smells) |
| CN2: | optic nerve (sees) |
| CN3, 4 and 6: | oculomotor, trochlear and abducens (moves eyes, constricts pupils, accommodates) |
| CN5: | trigeminal (chews and feels front of head) |
| CN7: | facial (moves the face, tastes, salivates and cries) |
| CN8: | acoustic (hears; regulates balance) |
| CN9: | glossopharyngeal (tastes, salivates, swallows, monitors carotid body and sinus) |
| CN10: | vagus (tastes, salivates, swallows, lifts palate) |
| CN11: | spinal accessory (turns head, lifts shoulders) |
| CN12: | hypoglossal (moves tongue). |

# The central nervous system

Consisting of the brain and spinal cord, the CNS is the body's central control system, receiving, integrating and interpreting all stimuli. The bony skull and vertebral column surround it.

The basic functional unit in the CNS is the neuron, down which travel chemically transmitted electrophysiological impulses. These impulses travels from the dendrite of the neuron, to the cell body and on to its axon. Impulses then pass to another neuron via a synapse.

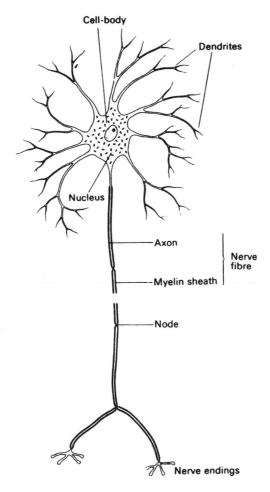

**Figure 1.2.** The neuron.

### Neurotransmission

There are as many as 100 billion individual neurons, each one connected to thousands of others. They are constantly communicating, sending up to 300 signals per second via synapses. An individual neuron can have up to 100,000 synapses, tiny gaps crossed by neurotransmitters, which cause an electrical change when they arrive. The number of possible routes for nerve signals is enormous and the permutations difficult to imagine.

Once an action potential or 'message' arrives at the nerve endings, calcium ions pass into it from extracellular fluid; the transmission is then emitted into the synaptic cleft and unites with the post-synaptic neuron of the receiving nerve. The 'message' can be increased, reduced, influenced or obliterated.

There are four main groups of neurotransmitters:

- Amines, such as acetylcholine, noradrenaline, dopamine and seratonin.
- Amino acids, such as glutamic acid and GABA (gamma aminobutyric acid).
- Purines, such as ATP (adenosine triphosphate).
- Peptides, such as enkephalins and endorphins.

## The brain

The transient period of brain growth in the human foetus is known as the growth spurt, during which time various cellular systems in the brain develop in a predetermined order and in relation to the growth spurt of the whole brain. Two main areas of brain development occur, the first concerning the order in which general areas of the brain develop, and the second, the order in which body localization advances within these areas. At birth, the brain weighs about 25% of its adult weight, and by 18 months it has reached 75%; this rapid growth slows down and it takes a further eight years for the brain to reach 95% of the total adult weight. (The adult brain weighs about 1,400 g, approximately 2% of total body weight.) Different parts of the brain grow at different rates and reach their maximum velocity at different times (May and Carter, 1995). With this extraordinary amount of activity occurring, it is surely surprising that more congenital abnormalities do not occur in the human baby.

The efficiency of the CNS increases with maturity and is closely associated with the process of learning; the more frequently used neuronal pathways become strengthened and preserved and may eventually become well established (Russell and Denver, 1975). This process may explain why rehabilitation and adaptation is greater in the young child following trauma, illness or congenital abnormality involving the CNS, than in the adult patient.

The brain has three major areas: the brain stem, the cerebellum and the cerebrum.

The brain stem is divided into the mid brain, pons and medulla.

The mid brain serves as the pathway between the cerebral hemispheres and the lower brain. It is the centre for auditory and visual reflexes. It contains the aqueduct of Sylvius and cranial nerves III and IV are located within it.

The pons (which is Latin for bridge) contains bands of transverse fibres connecting the mid brain and the medulla; many pathways pass through the pons, including the spinothalamic tracts, the corticospinal tracts and part of the reticular activating system; the pons contains the fourth

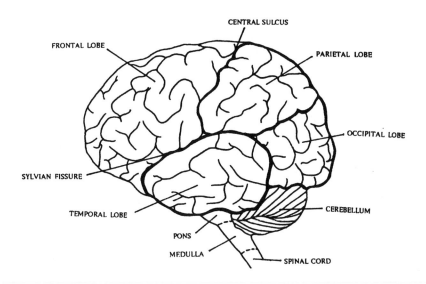

**Figure 1.3.** The brain stem.

ventricle and it also has some control over respiratory function. Cranial nerves 5 to 8 are situated within the pons.

The medulla also contains part of the fourth ventricle, sensory and motor tracts, cardiac, respiratory and vasomotor centres. Cranial nerves 9 to 11 exit from the medulla.

### The cerebrum

According to Nathan (1997) the cerebrum is not essential for life. He suggests that it is an added feature, appearing late in the evolution process and that all essential functions have been built into earlier models, millions of years previously. The cerebrum does, however, have a vast range of functions, which include the ability to learn, remember and store the individuals' unique experiences. The two cerebral hemispheres have slightly different functions and many studies have been performed to determine right- and left-sided functions and dominance. Our bodies are symmetrical, so a brain built on this double plan could risk functioning as two separate and uncoordinated organs; to overcome this, the two halves are connected by commissures throughout the spinal cord, hindbrain and mid brain. A thick band of fibres known as the corpus callosum connects each part of one hemisphere to the corresponding part in the other. At birth, both hemispheres have an equal capacity for development, but as the child grows, one hemisphere grows rapidly in relation to the other. Generally speaking, the right hemisphere appears more involved with spatial awareness, non-verbal ideas and thought processes; the left side appears more concerned with analytical thought processes and language. Nathan (1997) describes the left cerebral cortex as seeing the trees but not much of the forest, whereas the right side sees the forest but not too many of the trees! Left cerebral dominance is found in 90% of the population and these people are right handed; surprisingly, most, but not all, left-handed people also have a dominant left hemisphere.

The grey convoluted cortex of the cerebral hemispheres contains about 50 billion neurons and 250 billion glial cells. The grooves between each convolution or gyrus are called sulci or fissures; the advantage of having many sulci and fissures is that the surface area of the cortex is greatly increased. The underlying white matter consists of interconnecting groups of axons: one group extends from the cortex to other cortical areas of the same and opposite hemisphere, or to the brain stem, thalamus, basal ganglia or spinal cord; the other group extends from the thalamus to the cortex.

The white matter of the cortex contains three types of fibres: association fibres that link one area of cortex to another in the same hemisphere; commissural fibres (including the corpus callosum) that link the two cerebral hemispheres; and projection fibres which link one cerebral hemisphere to other parts of the brain, such as the basal ganglia. The paired basal ganglia are situated beneath the white matter of each cerebral hemisphere; these nuclei relay information from the cerebral cortex back to the motor cortex of the cerebrum, thus assisting in muscle co-ordination.

Each cerebral hemisphere is divided into lobes. The following gives a brief overview of these:

- The frontal lobe. The frontal lobe has two main functions: one is the motor control of voluntary movements, and the second is responsibility for emotional expression; the frontal eye field and Broca's speech area are both located in this lobe.
- The parietal lobe. The parietal lobe processes information necessary to create an awareness of the body and its relation to the external environment; it is concerned with the evaluation of all the general senses (and receives information from receptors in the skin, organs outside the CNS, muscles and joints); it is responsible for the evaluation of taste.
- The temporal lobe. The temporal lobe is the primary auditory receptive area and contains Wernicke's area (usually found in the dominant hemisphere and when damaged, is associated with fluent aphasia – words that are heard but not understood). The temporal lobe is the primary receptive area for hearing and receives information from both

ears, but mainly from the opposite one. The temporal lobe is also associated with equilibrium and, to a certain degree, memory and emotion.

- The occipital lobe. The occipital lobe is the primary visual cortex, controlling visual reflexes, perception and involuntary, smooth eye movements.

Although it is customary to divide the cerebral cortex into sensory and motor areas, the two kinds of areas are in fact, mainly mixed. The cortical areas are all connected in a two-way system with the thalamus. The diencephalon is a major division of the cerebrum and is divided into four regions: the thalamus, subthalamus, epithalamus and the hypothalamus.

**The thalamus**

The thalamus consists of a pair of egg-shaped masses of grey matter, situated deep within the centre of the hemispheres. It has connections to multiple areas of the brain. All sensory pathways (with the exception of the olfactory pathways) have both afferent and efferent connections with the thalamus. The thalamus is the last 'station' where impulses are processed before passing down to the cortex of the cerebrum. The thalamus is associated with the reticular activating system, the limbic system, attention and with conscious pain awareness.

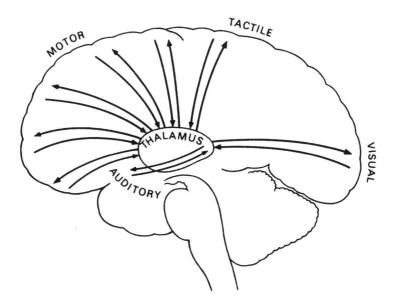

**Figure 1.4.** The thalamus.

## The subthalamus

The subthalamus is situated below the thalamus and is functionally related to the basal ganglia.

## The basal ganglia

The basal ganglia are the subcortical nuclei located deep within the cerebral hemispheres and are closely related functionally to the thalamus, subthalamus, substantia nigra and red nucleus. They form the motor control for fine body movements, particularly of the hands and lower extremities.

## The pineal gland

The epithalamus is composed of the pineal gland/body; this pea-sized body is situated at the posterior end of the third ventricle. Also known as the 'neuroendocrine transducer', this gland converts a signal received through the central nervous system (dark and light for example), into an endocrine signal (shifting the levels of hormone secretion). The pineal gland is associated with reception of light and dark sensation (the pineal gland in birds, for example, is proportionally large, particularly in migrating birds). The pineal gland secretes melatonin (derived from seratonin) – the amount of melatonin secretion is dictated by dark and inhibited by light; melatonin causes drowsiness and there is some speculation that the pineal gland is associated with seasonal affective disorder, including lack of energy, mood swings and depression.

## The hypothalamus and the autonomic nervous system (ANS)

The hypothalamus is the control centre for the autonomic nervous system and the neuroendocrine system. It forms part of the walls of the third ventricle and is situated in the basal region of the diencephalon. Many circuits connect the hypothalamus with areas such as the cerebral cortex, brain stem and thalamus. The optic chiasma crosses the floor of the hypothalamus, and the olfactory system is also adjacent and interconnected.

The ANS is split into the sympathetic nervous system, which could be viewed as catabolic, expending energy, for example in the 'fight or flight' mechanism, and the parasympathetic nervous system, which could be viewed as anabolic, conserving energy. As the centre for the autonomic nervous system, the hypothalamus has many essential functions; temperature regulation by monitoring blood temperature and sending efferent impulses to sweat glands, peripheral vessels and muscles, for example; it is associated with wakefulness and sleep cycles, visible physical expressions in response to emotions (such as blushing, clamminess), hypophysial secretions (growth hormone and follicle-stimulating hormone) and it is responsible for the hugely important task of regulating the visceral and somatic activities of the autonomic nervous system (heart rate, peristalsis, pupillary constriction and dilatation).

### The pituitary gland (or hypophysis)

The pituitary gland is connected to the hypothalamus by the pituitary stalk. The two lobes of the pituitary gland are the anterior and posterior lobes; the latter controls the secretion of vasopressin (antidiuretic hormone) and oxytocin; the former controls six major hormones relating to metabolic functioning: adrenocorticotrophic hormone (ACTH); thyroid stimulating hormone (TSH); follicle stimulating hormone (FSH), growth stimulating hormone (GSH), luteinizing hormone (LH) and prolactin. Feedback systems from afferent fibres in the hypothalamus (and consequently the pituitary), as well as from the target organ, help regulate the level of the various hormones.

### The internal capsule

The many nerve fibres from various parts of the cortex converge at the brain stem. As the fibres arrive at the thalamus/hypothalamus region, they are collectively called the internal capsule. They consist of a massive bundle of sensory and motor nerves connecting the various subdivisions of the brain and spinal cord. The afferent sensory fibres pass from the brain stem to the thalamus, to the internal capsule and on to the cerebral cortex; all efferent motor fibres leaving the cortex pass from the cortex to the internal capsule and then to the brain stem.

### The cerebellum

Located in the posterior fossa, the cerebellum is attached to the pons, medulla and mid brain by three paired cerebellar peduncles. These peduncles receive direct input from the spinal cord and brain stem and convey it to the cerebellar cortex and nuclei. The resulting excitory and inhibitory effects directly influence the motor system. There are many feedback loops in which cerebellar function is central to the maintenance of muscle activity, receiving and transmitting impulses. The cerebellum controls fine movement and co-ordinates muscle groups.

# Special systems within the brain

### The limbic system

In 1878, Paul Broca proposed that another lobe should be recognized; the lobe was not an obvious entity, but was spread throughout different parts of the brain. Since some of it surrounded the brain stem he named it the limbic lobe (*limbus* is Latin for border). It consists of the hippocampus, the amygdala and the cingulate gyrus.

The limbic system has come a long way over the millions of years since its olfactory origins, and is now responsible for adapting behaviour to situations in which we find ourselves. Connected to the hypothalamus, the septal area, the brain stem and to the reticular formation, the limbic lobe is constantly in touch with the outside world. With its rapid connections to the autonomic nervous system, the limbic lobe assists in controlling basic instinctual and emotional drives; it is also associated with short-term memory. The emotional responses are expressed through behavioural reactions, along with endocrine, somatic and visceral responses.

### The reticular activating system (RAS)

This diffuse system controls the sleep/wakefulness cycle and extends from the brain stem to the cerebral cortex. Stimulation of the brain stem

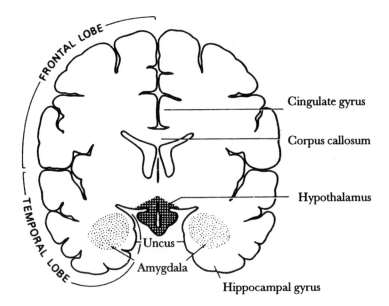

**Figure 1.5.** The limbic system.

portion of the RAS results in activation of the entire brain; stimulation of the thalamic portion causes generalized activity of the cerebrum, selective areas playing a role in the direction of attention to certain mental activities.

## The reticular formation

A group of neurons known collectively as the reticular formation are found within the brain stem and part of the diencephalon. The function of these neurons is to provide continuous impulse input to the muscles supporting the body against gravity and, in addition, to provide more general information about muscle activity.

## Cerebral blood flow

### The blood–brain barrier

There is a great need for homeostasis in the brain and it is consequently well protected against chemical imbalances. The structure of brain capillaries differs from capillaries in the rest of the body. The capillary walls around the body contain penetrable gaps that allow most substances to pass through. Those in the brain, however, have endothelial cells that are joined by tight junctions, which merge with the outer membrane layers of adjoining cells. These capillary walls make up the blood–brain barrier: all substances entering the brain from the blood must do so by active transport through the cell membranes or by diffusion through the endothelial cell membranes. Thus there is restriction of potentially harmful substances from entering the brain cells, while allowing nutrients to enter and excess substances to be removed. This process of selective permeability does cause difficulty when attempting to treat cerebral infections with antibiotics, or CNS tumours with chemotherapy agents. Although many breakthroughs have been accomplished, scientists are still struggling to find more effective ways to cross the blood–brain barrier.

### The physiology of cerebral blood flow (CBF)

About a fifth of the oxygen consumed by the body is used for the oxidation of glucose to provide energy. The brain is totally dependent on glucose for its metabolism (it has no glucose stores) and a lack of oxygen to the brain will result in irreversible brain damage. In normal conditions, blood flow rates to specific areas of the brain correlate directly with the metabolism of the cerebral tissue.

There are five physiological factors that can affect CBF in the normal brain. These include autoregulation and cerebral perfusion pressure (CPP), arterial oxygen tension (PaO$_2$), arterial blood carbon dioxide tension (PaCO$_2$), regional metabolic demand, and the autonomic nervous system. The interrelationships between these factors are many and complex. The property of the intracranial bed to allow a constant CBF in the face of a changing CPP is known as autoregulation, and the blood vessel diameter varies in response to transmural pressure changes and tissue metabolite accumulation. The CPP can be regarded as the difference between the mean arterial pressure (MAP) and the intracranial pressure (ICP). Hence CPP = MAP – ICP.

Above and below the normal limits of autoregulation, the CBF is directly related to the CPP and any disturbance to the CPP will cause damage. An acute sustained rise in CPP can cause disruption to the blood–brain barrier, oedema and ischaemia; a low CPP can cause tissue hypoxia and acidosis. Damage to the brain tissue itself, in the form of a tumour or head trauma, can abolish autoregulation in the affected area, and CBF then becomes directly dependent on CPP.

Changes in PaO$_2$ (arterial oxygen level) and PaCO$_2$ (arterial carbon dioxide level) directly affect the vascularity of the blood vessels and work in close combination with the autoregulation system described above; variations, particularly with regard to PaCO$_2$, can have catastrophic effects on CBF.

Cerebral blood flow has a direct relationship with cerebral metabolic activity: local increases in cerebral activity, for example during a seizure, provoke a simultaneous increase in CBF.

Cerebral blood vessels are innervated by parasympathetic, sympathetic and sensory nerves, although these factors do not appear to exert a major influence on CBF in normal circumstances.

## The cerebral arteries

The brain is supplied by two pairs of arteries, two internal carotid and two vertebral arteries. Cerebral circulation is divided into anterior and posterior circulation: the former includes the carotids, the middle cerebral and the anterior cerebral arteries; the latter includes the vertebral, basilar and posterior arteries.

The circle of Willis is the central, complex system of arteries, found at the base of the skull. It is little more than one square inch in diameter but, despite its size, the circle of Willis permits adequate blood supplies to reach all parts of the brain, even after one or more of the four arteries supplying it have been ligated.

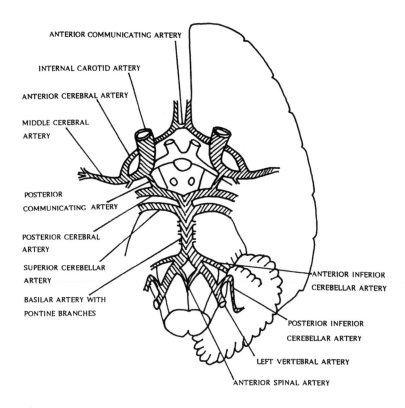

**Figure 1.6.** The circle of Willis.

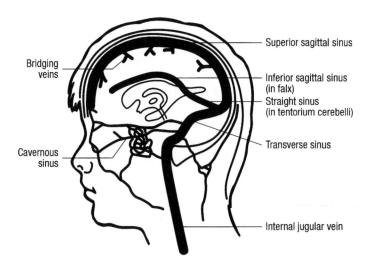

**Figure 1.7.** The main cerebral veins.

*The veins*

Unlike other arteries of the body which have corresponding veins, the circle of Willis has no female counterpart. Three main sinuses deserve recognition: first, the sagittal sinus into which the cerebral spinal fluid drains; second, the cavernous sinus into which venous blood from the eye drains – there are many important structures running by or through the cavernous sinus, including all the nerves entering the orbit, and the carotid artery – the third sinus is the transverse sinus, which runs close to the ear and may be involved in inner-ear infections. The veins and sinuses of the brain are unique in that they have no valves.

The veins of the brain drain into the internal jugular vein.

The brain is separated from the skull by the meninges – the pia, arachnoid and dura membranes. The meninges are supplied with blood by the anterior, middle and posterior arteries.

The thin and vascular pia mata sits against the brain. The arachnoid mata is avascular and separates the pia and dura mata. The dura lies up against the skull and this thick, double layer of connective tissue contains venous channels known as sinuses that lie between its two layers. The meninges cover the entire CNS including the spinal cord and the optic nerve.

## The ventricular system

Cerebrospinal fluid (CSF) is formed continuously by the vascular choroid plexus of the third ventricle and, in smaller amounts, in the third and fourth ventricles; a small amount is produced by the brain parenchyma.

Cerebrospinal fluid is a clear, colourless liquid and its function is twofold: first it provides buoyancy for the brain and second it helps maintain homeostasis by assisting in the control of the chemical environment of the CNS. It does this by conveying excessive components and unwanted substances away from the extracellular fluid and into the venous system. Cerebrospinal fluid moves from the lateral ventricles to the third and fourth ventricles and then to the subarachnoid space where it is reabsorbed via the arachnoid villi. Cerebrospinal fluid also flows down the spinal cord to the cisterns. The largest cistern is the lumbar cistern and is situated between L2 and S2. This is consequently the area where lumbar punctures are performed.

The total volume of CSF is formed and renewed about three times a day. The CSF volume in the ventricles is approximately 3.5 ml/kg and the turnover rate is about 5% of its total volume per minute. Marshall et al. (1990) suggest that the amounts produced in children are as yet undetermined. Waring and Jeansonne (1982), however, suggest that a child has 504 ml of CSF in the ventricles at any one time.

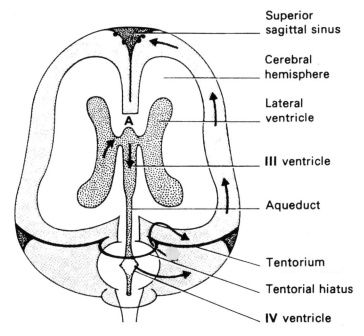

Superior
sagittal sinus

Cerebral
hemisphere

Lateral
ventricle

III ventricle

Aqueduct

Tentorium

Tentorial hiatus

IV ventricle

**Figure 1.8.** The ventricles.

## Intracranial elastance

The direct relationship between the intracranial compartments and cerebral dynamics is known as the principle of Munro. An increase in one compartment of the brain will cause a rise in ICP unless there is compensation in another compartment (brain elastance). Although acute rises in ICP due to coughing and sneezing for example, cause little disruption, pathological rises in brain volume will cause a malignant rise in ICP. Once a certain level is reached, compensation no longer occurs and small increases in volume will cause major increases in ICP. Brain herniation will then occur and this can be intracranial, transtentorial, tonsillar or cingulate.

## The spinal cord

The spinal cord contains inner grey and outer white matter; the former contains neuronal cell bodies and synapses; the latter contains ascending pathways that relay sensory information to the brain, and descending pathways that relay motor information away from the brain. There are three main sensory systems entering the spinal cord: pain/temperature, proprioception (the ability to sense the position of the limbs and their movements with eyes closed) and light touch. The pathway for pain and temperature enters the spinal cord and almost immediately crosses over, ascends to the thalamus on the opposite side and on to the cerebral cortex; hence a lesion of the spinothalamic tract will result in the loss of these sensations, below the level of the lesion. The pathway for proprioception initially remains on the same side of the spinal cord that it enters; it crosses over at the junction between the spinal cord and the brain stem; hence any injury to the posterior column results in a disturbance to proprioception, ipsilateral below the level of the lesion. The pathway for light touch combines both features of the above two pathways and hence remains intact in cases of ipsilateral cord lesions.

The motor (corticospinal) pathway extends from the cerebral cortex, down through the brain stem and crosses over at the junction of the spinal cord and the brain stem. Motor neuron disturbance above the corticospinal pathway synapse is termed an upper motor neuron defect, and that below as a lower motor neuron defect.

## The spine

The spinal cord is surrounded by the 26 spinal vertebrae. The vertebrae are stacked one on top of the other to support the head and spine, and form a flexible column. The adult vertebral column consists of seven cervical vertebrae, 12 thoracic, five lumbar, one sacral (five fused) and one coccygeal (three fused) vertebrae. The first cervical vertebra is known as the atlas because it supports the head, as the Greek god Atlas supported the heavens on his shoulders. The atlas allows the nodding motion of the head. The second cervical vertebra is known as the axis, because it forms a pivot point for the atlas to move the skull in a twisting motion. The pivot is a peglike protrusion, which extends through the opening of the atlas and is known as the dens or odontoid process. Hanging or severe whiplash injury will cause direct pressure on this area, crushing the lower medulla and adjacent spinal cord, with resulting death.

The vertebral column is stabilized by muscles and ligaments that allow twisting and bending movements, while limiting potentially harmful movements that might cause damage to the spinal cord. The spinal column is the point of attachment for the muscles of the back. In addition, the column helps keep the body erect, provides support for the weight of the body, and its resilient intervertebral discs act as shock absorbers.

# The skull

The skull is the bony framework of the head and is composed of the eight bones of the cranium and the 14 bones of the face. The cranium encloses the brain and provides a protective vault. The bones of the skull are known as sutures; premature fusion of the skull sutures is known as craniosynostosis.

# Assessment of the neurosurgical child

Consciousness can be described as 'a general awareness of oneself and the surrounding environment' (Aucken and Crawford, 1999). It is estimated by the subjective observation of arousability and behaviour in response to stimuli (Ellis and Cavanagh, 1992); consistent assessment between observers is therefore difficult and, at times, unreliable.

Nurses are in a unique position to detect subtle changes in the child's neurology, as they are usually the most consistent carers; they should also use the mother's unique knowledge and understanding of her child, whenever appropriate. Formal neurological assessment should be undertaken in conjunction, and not instead of, general observation of the child; attention should be given to the child's surroundings, activities (such as playing, or lack of playing), and response to his or her mother.

All professionals caring for the child should watch for potential or anticipated changes in the child's condition. A delay in identifying and acting upon changes can have a direct relationship on subsequent management and outcomes.

Various coma charts have been devised, mainly based on the Glasgow coma chart, in an attempt to standardize clinical assessment of consciousness.

The Glasgow Coma Scale (GCS) was devised by Jennet and Teasdale (1974). The scale is divided into three categories comprising eye opening, best verbal response and best motor response; each category is further divided and the resulting graph provides a visual record of the improvement or deterioration of the patient's neurological status. The resulting numerical score is used in conjunction with the patient's vital signs in identifying the patient's status and any necessary nursing and medical interventions.

The GCS is difficult to apply to children in its present form because many of the responses required involve an adult neurodevelopmental function, in particular the development of language and the ability to

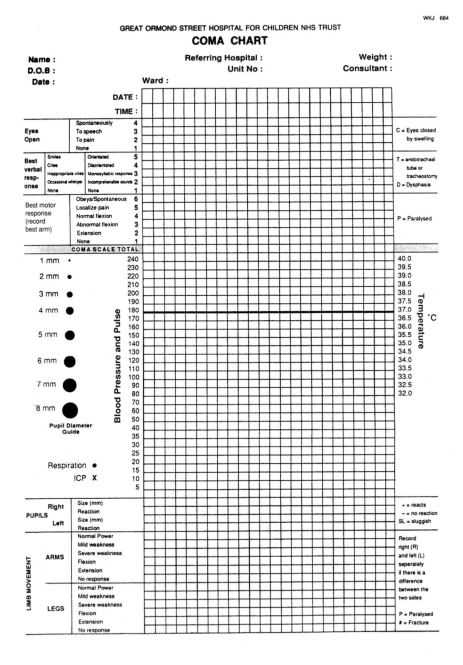

**Figure 1.9.** A paediatric coma chart.

localize to pain. Many centres have developed their own charts adapted specifically to children. The Paediatric Neurosurgical Benchmarking group in the UK has spent much time discussing the various problems surrounding a specific chart for children, encompassing the developmental and chronological ages of children. Whatever chart is used, appropriate education in its use is just as important as the chart itself; written, verbal and visual education methods (such as a video) can be employed, highlighting issues such as how to interpret and score a neonate's neurological status, or how to assess a child with severe neurodevelopmental delay.

It should be remembered when assessing children that regression may occur due to hospitalization, separation from their parents and home environment, and the impact of the illness itself (May and Carter, 1995).

Further information concerning the use of paediatric coma scoring and education may be found in Simpson and Reilley (1982), Raimondi and Hirschner (1984), Morray et al. (1984). An education video regarding coma scoring in young children, can be obtained from the department of illustration at the Great Ormond Street Hospital for Sick Children NHS Trust, Great Ormond Street, London WC1N 3JH.

## Raised intracranial pressure

The normal range of intracranial pressure is between 0–15 mm Hg in adults and 0–8 mm Hg in infants (James, 1989). Raised intracranial pressure may result directly from a space-occupying lesion such as a tumour or a haematoma, from cerebral oedema, or due to the presence of hydrocephalus. Typical signs include headache (classically, early morning headache), vomiting and papilloedema (papilloedema will not occur in the baby as his head circumference will expand to compensate). Visual deterioration can be a sign of chronic raised intracranial pressure.

Changes in vital signs are a late indicator of acute raised intracranial pressure in children, and irritability, drowsiness and pupil dilatation with a decreased reaction to light, are earlier indicators of neurological deterioration.

## Headache

The intracranial structures that are sensitive to pain are the middle meningeal arteries and branches, the venous sinuses and the large arteries and the dura at the base of the brain, all of which have a rich sensory innervation. In the presence of raised intracranial pressure the cerebral vessels dilate in an attempt to provide an adequate blood supply to the brain. Dilatation of the vessels, traction on the bridging veins and stretching of the arteries at the base of the brain, cause a headache. These headaches do not usually show any particular localization towards the site of a specific lesion, but are often noted to be frontal or occipital.

Early morning headache associated with raised intracranial pressure occurs as a result of an additional rise of this pressure during rapid-eye-movement (REM) sleep. During REM (*paradoxical*) sleep, the heart and respiratory rate are increased, movements of hands and toes occur, and movements involving the whole body such as turning over, take place. The resulting increased metabolic rate and carbon dioxide production causes hypercapnia and vasodilation – hence the headache. Early morning headaches should always be thought of as organic in cause.

### Vomiting

The areas of the brain associated with vomiting are the vagal motor centres located in the floor of the fourth ventricle and consequently any lesion involving this area will be associated with vomiting. The vagal motor centre also mediates the motility of the gastrointestinal tract – slow gastric emptying is often associated with raised intracranial pressure.

Any distortion of the brain stem as a result of raised intracranial pressure will result in vomiting. If a lesion directly affects the vomiting mechanism, the afferent limb is short-circuited and vomiting occurs without nausea – with resulting forceful or projectile vomiting.

### Papilloedema

The subdural and subarachnoid spaces continue along the optic nerve, and therefore increased pressure within the cranium is transmitted along the nerve. The resulting oedema of the nerve, in particular the nerve head, can be visualized as a blurring of the optic disc, along with enlargement of the retinal veins with absence of their pulsations. If the situation continues, atrophy of the nerve head occurs with a decline in visual acuity, followed by blindness.

Depending on the circumstances, papilloedema may be quite a late finding with raised intracranial pressure and, indeed, is not present in every patient with raised pressure.

### Drowsiness

Raised intracranial pressure causes impairment of the reticular activating system, causing drowsiness; this will continue to coma and death if the pressure is unrelieved.

# Changes in vital signs

### Pulse

The pulse is relatively stable during the early stages of raised intracranial pressure, particularly in the young child. Bradycardia is controlled by pressure on the vagal mechanism in the medulla and is a compensatory mechanism to force blood upwards into the engorged brain. If the pressure is not relieved, the pulse becomes thready and irregular and finally stops.

### Respiration

As consciousness declines, the cerebral cortex becomes suppressed more readily than the brain stem and, in the adult patient, a change in respiration will normally follow a decrease in the level of consciousness. Alterations in the respiratory pattern are due to direct pressure on the brain stem. In the infant, respiratory irregularity and increasing apnoea attacks are often among the early symptoms of excessively raised intracranial pressure and can rapidly lead to respiratory arrest.

Acute pulmonary oedema can occur in any age group following a sudden rise in intracranial pressure, requiring the need for ventilatory support. Pulmonary oedema is a very serious complication that may result in death.

### Blood pressure

Blood pressure and pulse remain relatively stable in the early stages of raised intracranial pressure, particularly in the infant.

As intracranial pressure increases, the blood pressure rises reflexively to compensate; Cushing's response results, with a rise in blood pressure, a drop in pulse and a variation in respiratory pattern. With continued deterioration, the blood pressure starts to drop. As previously mentioned, Cushing's response is a late finding in children with raised intracranial pressure.

### Temperature

During the compensatory phase of increasing intracranial pressure, the temperature will remain stable; during the decompensatory change high temperatures may occur due to hypothalamic dysfunction, or oedema to the connecting tracts.

**Pupil reaction**

The oculomotor nerve (III) controls pupillary function. Pupils should be examined for size, shape and equality; when compared with each other, the pupils should be equal in size. Normally, pupillary constriction is brisk, although pupils in younger people tend to be larger and more responsive to light; withdrawal of light should result in pupillary dilation. In addition to the constriction of the pupil that occurs with direct light stimulation (known as the direct light response) there is a weaker constriction of the non-stimulated pupil (known as the consensual light reflex). This occurs as a result of fibres that cross the optic chiasma and the posterior commisure of the mid brain. Parasympathetic fibres cause contraction of the pupilloconstrictor fibres of the iris, causing the pupils to contract. Sympathetic fibres cause the pupillodilator muscles to dilate.

Sluggish pupillary reaction is found in conditions that cause some compression of the oculomotor nerve, such as cerebral oedema or a cerebral lesion. Further, oculomotor nerve compression causes a downward pressure, trapping the oculomotor nerve between the tentorium and the herniating temporal lobe and resulting in fixed, dilated pupils. Should both pupils be in a mid position and non reactive, neither sympathetic nor sympathetic innervation is operational; this is usually associated with severe anoxia, midbrain infarction or transtentorial herniation, and consequently, death. Atropine-like drugs will cause dilated pupils, so this possibility must be taken into account.

Very small, pinpoint, non-reactive pupils indicate damage to the pons, which controls many motor pathways and vital functions, and is consequently a very grave sign. Opiate drugs can also cause this reaction and should be considered in the overall assessment of the patient.

**Brain herniation**

If increased intracranial pressure is present in only one compartment of the brain, there is a tendency for the brain that shares that component to be squeezed towards another compartment of lower pressure. The two main brain herniations are downward through the foramen magnum and downward through the tentorial hiatus. The latter, also known as uncal herniation, occurs when one cerebral hemisphere expands in mass; the oculomotor nerve, mid brain and posterior cerebral arteries run through the uncus; the result is that the pupil on the side of the lesion will become fixed and dilated (pressure on the nerve reduces the constrictor effect on the pupil and the dilator effects of the sympathetic nerves take over); pressure on the reticular apparatus causes drowsiness; finally, compression of the posterior cerebral arteries produces ischaemia and possible infarction of the occipital cortex.

Foramen magnum herniation occurs when compressive lesions of the posterior fossa push those structures nearest it, down towards the cervical canal – in particular the cerebellar tonsils. The resulting pressure on the brain stem causes respiratory disturbance, but minimal alteration in the level of consciousness as the compression is below the level of the reticular activating system. Death will rapidly follow if the intracranial pressure is not rapidly relieved.

# Clinical neuroimaging

## X-rays

Despite CT and MRI scanning, X-rays are still a valuable diagnostic tool in the diagnosis of skull fractures, abnormal skull formations and spinal fractures. Abnormal calcification can be identified by X-ray in specific brain tumours such as craniopharyngiomas and some pineal tumours.

## CT scan

Computerized tomography is now widely available, although it has reduced sensitivity in detecting lesions adjacent to bone, or small soft tissue lesions. Narrow X-ray beams are passed through the body and are absorbed or transmitted, depending on the density of the tissue. The transmitted information is detected by an array of scanners, which convert it into light photons, in direct proportion to its intensity and energy. The photons are converted into electrical signals, digitized on a computer and manipulated to reproduce images. Brain tissue appears as a grey shade, CSF as darker and air as black. Bone appears white. Intravenous contrast enhancement improves anatomical detail. The disadvantage of repeated CT scanning is that it is radioactive, and cranial ultrasound is preferable in the early days for the infant with hydrocephalus who may require several scans during his life.

## Cranial ultrasound

A probe is moved around the anterior fontanelle of the baby and through this, high frequency, pulsed sound waves are transmitted; the reception and recording of these sound waves are transmitted back to a receiver. Different body tissues will impede or absorb sound waves in a different way and the resulting images can be used to evaluate the dimensions of the ventricles. Regular images of the ventricles can thus be obtained without the need for a CT scan, and the technique is frequently used in neonatal and special care baby units.

## Magnetic resonance imaging (MRI)

The patient is placed within the scanner, and this may require sedation or general anaesthesia in some children. The nuclei of hydrogen atoms in tissues are aligned through the use of a strong magnetic field. Radio-frequency waves are then applied, which sets the nuclei rotating on their axes in a uniform manner; as they return to their normal alignment, they give off tiny radio-frequency signals and these are converted and analysed on a computer. By using a particular pulse frequency, images known as T1 and T2 can be obtained: T1 images are specifically used to define anatomy and T2 images are used to define soft tissues. If a contrast medium is utilized, T1 images are used, as contrast enhancement is not detected on T2 sequences.

Images obtained from MRI scanning are far superior to those obtained from CT, but the costs involved mean that it is not readily available in all centres.

It is now possible for surgeons to use the MRI scan taken preoperatively, to guide them during the operation itself. Once the head is immobilised at the time of surgery, a computerized image guidance system is used to co-register anatomical landmarks visible on the patient (for example, the eyes and ears), with the corresponding features on the scan image. The surgeon can then use a pointing device to orient the operative field, with respect to the brain pictures. This imaging is currently known as 'Wand' sequencing.

## Single photon emission computerized tomography (SPECT)

This technique uses a rotating gamma camera. Physiological imaging studies are obtained that measure blood perfusion of the brain. It is being increasingly used for children undergoing investigations into intractable epilepsy; it can also discriminate between tumour recurrence and radiation necrosis.

## Positive emission tomography (PET)

Few centres can offer a PET scan due to the huge expense of the required cyclotron unit. The scan also produces poor anatomical detail. It is used to study regional blood flow and to measure regional physiological functions such as glucose and oxygen uptake and metabolism.

## Cerebral angiography

This procedure is usually performed under general anaesthesia in children. Contrast medium is injected intravenously and images of the child's blood vessels are obtained. It is mainly used for the detection of vascular abnormalities and the displacement of cerebral vessels by tumours.

## Suggested texts for further reading

Carola R, Harley JP, Noback CR (1990) Human Anatomy and Physiology. International edn. New York: McGraw-Hill.
Goldberg S (1997) Clinical Neuroanatomy Made Ridiculously Simple. Miami FL: MedMaster Inc.
Nathan P (1988) The Nervous System. London: Whurr.
Hickey J (1997) Neurological and Neurosurgical Nursing. Philadelphia PA: Lippincott-Raven.

## References

Aucken S, Crawford B (1999) Neurological assessment. In Guerrero D (ed.) Neuro Oncology for Nurses. London: Whurr, p. 62.
Hickey JV (ed.) (1992) The Clinical Practice of Neurologial and Neuromedical Nursing. Philadelphia PA: Lippincott & Co.
Ellis A, Cavanagh S (1992) Aspects of neurosurgical assessment using the Glasgow Coma Scale. Intensive and Critical Nursing Care 8: 94–9.
James HE (1989) Intracranial dynamics. In Nussbaum E (ed.) Pediatric Intensive Care. New York: Futura.
Jennet B, Teasdale G (1974) Assessment of coma and impaired consciousness. Lancet 2: 81–4.
May L, Carter B (1995) Nursing support and care: meeting the needs of the child and family with altered cerebral function In Carter B, Dearman A (eds) Child Health Care Nursing. Oxford: Blackwell Science, pp: 363–91.
Marshall SB, Marshall LF, Vos HR, Chestnut HM (1990) Neurosurgical Critical Care. Orlando FL: WB Saunders Co.
Morray JP, Tyler DC, Jones TK, Shintz JT, Lemire RJ (1984) Coma scale used for brain injured children. Critical Care Medicine 12: 1018–20.
Nathan P (1997) The Nervous System. London: Whurr, pp: 77–187.
Raimondi AJ, Hirschner J (1984) Head injury in the infant and toddler. Coma scoring and outcome scale. Child's Brain 11: 12–35.
Russell WR, Denver AJ (1975) Explaining the Brain, 15. Oxford: Oxford University Press.
Simpson D, Reilly P (1982) Paediatric Coma Scale. Lancet August, 450.
Waring WW, Jeansonne L (1982) Normal cerebrospinal fluid. In Waring WW, Jeansonne LO (eds) Practical Manual of Pediatrics. St Louis MO: Mosby.

# Chapter 2
# Hydrocephalus

## Introduction

Idiopathic hydrocephalus occurs at a rate of 0.48/1,000 live births
(El Shafer and El Rough, 1987). Hydrocephalus may also be the result
of intracranial infection or intraventricular haemorrhage, or secondary
to cerebral tumour. Hydrocephalus is caused by a disturbance in
CSF (cerebrospinal fluid) circulation, either due to a problem with
absorption ('communicating' hydrocephalus), or obstruction ('non-
communicating' hydrocephalus). The classic concept of hydrocephalus
is characterized by

- increased intracranial pressure;
- dilatation of the CSF pathways;
- increased CSF volume.

However, hydrocephalus is today being recognized as a multifocal disease
with a heterogeneous pathogenesis (Morn, 1995).

There are two main factors that determine the outcome of the child
with hydrocephalus. First, hydrocephalus affects the brain functionally
and morphologically. Neuronal development and myelination of the brain
are disturbed in varying degrees, depending on the time of onset of hydrocephalus – particularly in the foetal and infantile stages of development;
thus better outcomes should be obtained by shortening the time of
disease onset and the time of surgical treatment. Second, hydrocephalus
may be present concomitantly with primary brain damage, or it may
actually be caused by primary brain damage.

It is now apparent that progressive or prolonged enlargement of the
ventricles concurrent with only mild increases in intracranial pressure can
damage the brain (Del Bigio, 1993). The periventricular white matter in
patients with hydrocephalus is oedematous, has atonal damage and

demyelination, which may be permanent; the grey matter exhibits disori-
entation and dendritic deterioration, although most of these cells do not
die until the late stages of hydrocephalus. Cortical connectivity is
impaired, and diminished metabolism and membrane turnover has been
suggested during acute hydrocephalus (Del Bigio and McAllister, 1999).
Early intervention and treatment of hydrocephalus would therefore seem
beneficial, but might not reverse the above pathophysiological changes.

Morn (1993) produced the following factors that relate to intractable
hydrocephalus:

Factors related to patients:

* degree of hydrocephalus;
* associated malformations;
* brain damage due to primary disease;
* duration of hydrocephalus;
* causative disorders of hydrocephalus;
* others.

Factors related to management:

* time of diagnosis;
* time of onset of treatment;
* technical problems of shunting operations;
* problems of maintaining shunt function;
* shunt complications;
* others.

Some of these aspects will be elaborated upon later.

## Clinical evaluation

Diagnosis may occur *in utero,* but more commonly begins on first assessment and examination of the child. The typical appearance of a baby with
hydrocephalus includes increasing head circumference (which may be
noticed, for example, by parents, a health visitor, clinic doctor) and
bulging fontanelle; poor feeding or vomiting is also common; sunsetting
eyes, dilated scalp veins and drowsiness will follow if treatment does not
commence. The older child will display symptoms of headache and
vomiting, along with papilloedema, lethargy, poor school performance
and possible developmental delay.

The premature baby may have an ultrasound performed through the
anterior fontanelle, providing information as to the ratio of ventricular

size to cerebral cortex, and thus the diagnosis of hydrocephalus may be established.

The majority of babies/children will be referred from the community or from a local hospital; a CT scan will be performed, providing the diagnosis of hydrocephalus. During clinical examination, the head circumference will be measured and plotted alongside the baby's height and weight, to establish the ratio between them and which centiles the baby fits into; this will provide a baseline assessment for future measurements.

Following the diagnosis of hydrocephalus, there are treatment options to be considered. Insertion of a shunt may be the required treatment for the child with non-communicating hydrocephalus secondary to meningitis or of congenital origin. If an obstructive tumour is the cause, then tumour removal may sometimes alleviate the need for permanent CSF drainage; if the baby is very premature then temporary measures to control the CSF volume such as daily ventricular/spinal tapping may be necessary until the baby is fit enough for surgery. Insertion of a shunt remains the treatment for many babies and children with hydrocephalus, although the advent of ventriculostomy is revolutionizing the treatment for those with obstructive hydrocephalus.

Shunting will also be the treatment for those children with the rare congenital abnormality known as Dandy Walker syndrome. The clinical sequelae vary widely, but include posterior fossa cysts and hydrocephalus; developmental delay is common. Cystospinal fluid shunting is advocated and ventricular peritoneal shunting is sometimes also necessary.

## Preoperative care

Treatment begins on admission, by encouraging the family to participate in the care of their child and involving them in discussions and treatment plans. Giving birth to a baby with a congenital deformity will be a shock to parents. In addition, mother and her young baby may have been moved from their maternity hospital to the paediatric neurosurgical ward of another hospital, often not near home or relatives; the mother may feel frightened and isolated, and this can be partially relieved by a reassuring and informative approach from medical and nursing staff.

Once diagnosis has been established and a treatment plan discussed, the nurse can help prepare the parents for their baby's surgery by providing diagrammatic information, literature to read and the time to answer their questions. Introducing them to other families with hydrocephalic children may be helpful, although careful selection may be necessary to avoid introducing too many concerns about the more complex possible complications at this early stage!

The parents may wish to participate in the preoperative care of their child by bathing it prior to surgery and washing its hair (this may require a wash with hibiscus for example, in accordance with hospital guidelines). The play specialist will work with the family in preparing the older child psychologically for surgery, using the family's knowledge of the child and the child's own understanding of his hospitalization. Such issues as hair shaving, however minimal the shave, will need discussion and explanation. The anaesthetic itself may cause anxiety and misunderstanding. One young child was told by the anaesthetist that he would be 'put to sleep for the operation' and was unduly distressed following this conversation. He tearfully explained that his dog had recently been taken to the vets where he had been 'put to sleep' and had never since returned home; he therefore assumed the same fate was to happen to him. Good communication with the child will highlight and hopefully alleviate such misconceptions.

A paediatric physiotherapy assessment will highlight problems such as head and trunk control; advice can be given to parents with regard to the correct handling of their baby. Postural tone will be assessed and spasticity or flaccidity noted, particularly in those infants with a grade three or four intraventricular haemorrhage; baseline observations will assist the physiotherapist in working with this baby postoperatively. Many premature babies may by necessity have been nursed in positions not conducive to good head moulding or limb positioning. The physiotherapist and nurses must work together in teaching the parents correct positioning for their baby: greater midline orientation may be required, with the baby's legs supported in a central position rather than splayed apart – this can be achieved by providing a supportive 'nest' of bedclothes around the baby; this also provides a secure environment and the baby is less likely to suffer 'startle' reflexes and positioning. Regular repositioning of the infant should include the head to reduce the effects of moulding.

## Surgery for hydrocephalus

### Shunts

The parents may accompany their child to the anaesthetic room. Surgery will take approximately 45 minutes, but parents need to be aware that, with anaesthetic care and recovery, the child will be away from the ward for a longer period.

The aim of the shunt is to drain CSF from the ventricles to an extracranial part of the body, to be reabsorbed. The peritoneum remains the optimum choice as its membrane is highly permeable and will therefore absorb CSF easily. A ventricular-atrial shunt is used for children in whom the abdominal cavity is not appropriate, due, for example, to poor absorption following abdominal surgery, or where there may be an increased risk of infection due to the presence of a gastrostomy tube. A ventricular-atrial shunt may be difficult to insert in the premature infant who has had numerous previous central venous lines placed, and consequently a ventricular-pleural shunt might be necessary in these extreme cases.

## Postoperative care

The child's neurological status should be regularly assessed and any deterioration reported. Signs of overdrainage, such as a deeply depressed anterior fontanelle in the baby, extreme pallor, vomiting, tachycardia, hypotension and headache, indicate that it should be nursed flat and supported medically as necessary. Sudden low pressure in the neonate following shunt insertion can lead to respiratory depression and the baby may need oxygen or even bagging; laying the infant in the head down position should rapidly resolve the situation, although fluid resuscitation may occasionally be required. Signs of raised intracranial pressure, such as a persistently raised anterior fontanelle in the baby, possible bradycardia and hypertension, vomiting and headache, indicate inadequate shunting, which might be improved by nursing the child in the upright position. Signs of intraventricular haemorrhage, fortunately a rare occurrence following a shunt insertion, would include a deteriorating neurological status, with signs of both haemorrhage and shunt blockage. In this situation, the shunt may be removed and an external ventricular drain inserted. The outcome will be determined by the degree of haemorrhage.

Following a straightforward shunt insertion, the premature infant may require a greater degree of nursing and medical input due to a compromised respiratory system from previous ventilation; the infant may also be rendered cardiovascularly unstable due to the rapid change in intracranial pressure; he or she will require close monitoring, artificial warmth in the form of an incubator or baby therm, and intravenous fluids. Preparing parents for such possibilities will help alleviate anxiety, particularly because the parents will be familiar and experienced with the technology and equipment being used, but could see this as a backward step unless prepared for such possibilities.

The nurse will guide parents in participating in their child's care, assisting them with re-establishing feeding and handling the child in accordance with medical instructions (this will vary between hospitals; some children will be nursed flat for a period of hours/days and others will be handled normally immediately following surgery). Even the most experienced mother will initially be anxious during the immediate postoperative period and should be reassured that her confidence in handling and comforting her child remains important. Assessing her baby's fontanelle tension even at this early stage is a useful gauge of the effectiveness of the working shunt, and one that should be encouraged while under nursing guidance. The mother will thus begin to feel more confident with her baby's condition.

Intravenous fluids may be necessary while oral feeding is re-established. This may take a day or two in the small infant and plasma electrolytes should be checked along with a full blood count; even with minimal blood loss during surgery, the small baby in particular, may have acquired an abnormal blood profile that requires correction.

Analgesia should be administered regularly as prescribed, the tunnelling from the peritoneal catheter causing particular discomfort. Repositioning the child and encouraging neck movement, will help relieve the stiff neck that follows shunt insertion and which often tends to be a common source of discomfort in the days following surgery. Although uncomfortable in the immediate postoperative period, a baby's head can be supported by towels in the head-hugger position and gently turned regularly. There is no reason why postoperative infants should not be nursed intermittently on the shunt side, although with the very thin skin of the premature infant this may be for short periods only.

The method of wound closure will vary between units; it is customary to allow wound healing prior to bathing or hair washing; non-dissolvable sutures can be removed by the community team thus allowing earlier discharge and minimizing the disruption to the child and family.

## Complications

There are potential complications following insertion of a shunt.

### Blockage

The incidence of mechanical shunt malfunction is approximately 30% over one year, and peaks in the first few months after shunt placement; shunt occlusion is the most common shunt complication in paediatrics and constitutes 50% of all shunt complications (Detwiller et al., 1999). Shunt blockage can occur at any time and may be due to choroid plexus blocking the proximal tip of the catheter, or infection blocking the tip or distal end. Shunt blockage is a neurosurgical emergency and needs immediate attention, as the build up in intracranial pressure can cause neurological damage, and eventually death if left untreated. The length of time that an individual child can tolerate shunt blockage varies enormously between several hours and days, and this unpredictability means that each potential shunt blockage must be taken seriously. All or part of the shunt will need replacing if blocked.

### Overdrainage

This is now being recognized as an increasing problem and one that can be difficult to resolve. Subdural haematomas may occur as a direct result of overdrainage, causing further difficulties in treatment.

Slit ventricle syndrome (SVS) describes a longer term complication of overdrainage that occurs in approximately 1% of shunted paediatric patients (Epstein et al., 1988). The aetiology is unclear but has been attributed to overshunting, intracranial hypertension, periodic shunt malfunction and decreased intracranial compliance. The ventricles are small on CT scan, but the pressure within them can be very high. The child complains of headaches and, less frequently, vomiting. The low-pressure valve will consequently be changed to a medium or high-pressure resistance valve, or an antisyphon device. In extreme situations a subtemporal decompression craniectomy has been performed, with mixed results.

### Underdrainage

This results in enlarged ventricles and necessitates changing to a lower pressure valve.

### Infection

The majority of shunt infections are due to contamination at the time of surgery and consequently occur most commonly within three months of shunt insertion. Gram-positive organisms are the most common cause of infection in paediatrics, *staphylococcus epidermidis* being found in approximately 40% of shunt infections (Pople et al., 1992). Treatment for shunt infections varies between units, but usually consists of a course of intravenous and intrathecal antibiotics following removal of the infected shunt.

### External ventricular drainage (EVD) system

An external ventricular drainage system (EVD) is required during this treatment prior to insertion of a new shunt system once treatment is complete. This external system allows CSF to drain as determined by gravity – the height of the drainage chamber above the level of the child's ventricles controlling the amount of CSF drained. The correct position should be measured by drawing an imaginary line from the outside corner of the eye to the external auditory canal; the midpoint of this line is the location of the foramen of Munro and is the zero point for the EVD system.

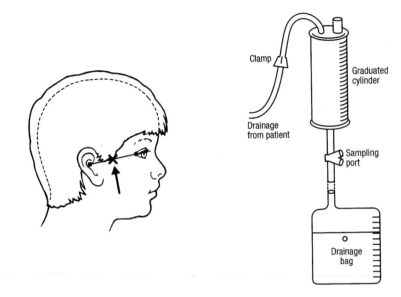

**Figure 2.1a.** Measurement for EVD.　　2.1b External ventricular drainage system.

The neurosurgeon will determine the desired amount of CSF drainage and hence the height of the drain. Appropriate nurse training and education is required for safe care of these systems (Terry and Nisbet, 1991; Birdsall and Greif, 1990). Thorough understanding is essential of the signs of overdrainage and underdrainage of CSF and the necessary action required (this may be as simple as the lowering or raising of the drain in accordance with medical instruction, to increase or decrease the amount of CSF drained). There is currently a system under study involving a transducer, which would enable the child on external ventricular drainage to move about freely without the involved remeasuring that is currently required. This would clearly be an advantage when caring for the active young child on drainage for many days.

The small child on external ventricular drainage may lose significant amounts of sodium in the CSF drained, as demonstrated by a drop in plasma sodium. Plasma electrolytes should be checked regularly for all children on EVD, and sodium supplements given intravenously or orally as required. Regular CSF samples should be obtained from the drainage system for analysis, and also to assess the levels of intrathecal antibiotics.

The child's care should be performed in a planned method to allow optimum time for more normal pastimes, such as sleep, play, schooling and rest, over the minimum treatment period of ten days.

A new shunt system will then be inserted on the opposite side of the head to the EVD, which will be removed.

## Discharge planning

Once a shunt has been inserted and the child has recovered sufficiently to be discharged from the neurosurgical unit, the parents need to feel confident in the care of their child. This requires educating them with regard to shunt dysfunction and the required treatment should this occur. Many childhood illnesses mimic the signs of shunt blockage – headaches and vomiting being among the commonest. The ward nurse and clinical nurse specialist, if available, are crucial people in this education process, ensuring that each family is familiar with the signs and symptoms of shunt dysfunction. Findings from a study by Stanton (1987) indicate that nurses see themselves as the primary educators of parents. Neuroscience nurses must not only provide clinical and disease information but must also ensure that parents are aware when to seek appropriate medical intervention (Kirk et al., 1992). This information is crucial and even life saving. To ensure that parents have read and understood written information given by the ward and discussed the issues surrounding their child's shunt, they may be asked to sign a form to confirm that this education has taken place. In the light of growing litigation in medicine today, this would seem a logical procedure.

Once home, parents must be encouraged to contact their general practitioner, local hospital or neurosurgical unit at the earliest opportunity should their child become unwell. Discharge home following insertion of a first shunt is an anxious time for the family and in particular for the mother, who will probably be the main carer. The responsibility often seems awesome, and an approachable doctor or nurse in hospital and in the community can help to reassure parents. Effective communication between all members of the multidisciplinary team and the community is essential, ensuring that the local hospital and GP are informed of the child's treatment and discharge. The ward physiotherapist will contact the community physiotherapist should the child have ongoing needs. Those children more seriously affected may benefit from a neurodevelopmental assessment and programme once fully recovered from surgery.

Schoolteachers and any other main carers of children with hydrocephalus must be aware of potential complications and what to do/who to contact should the child become unwell. Booklets relating to hydrocephalus and the possible complications should be available for the community team as well as to parents, to assist in this education process.

Should a clinical nurse specialist in neurosurgery be available she or he is clearly the ideal person to co-ordinate with the community regarding rehabilitation needs, social service requirements, continuing education and the relaying of information (Guin, 1995). The more secure and confident the family feels within the community setting, the better it will deal with any problems arising.

# Ventriculostomy

Neuroendoscopy was created in 1920 by a urologist who succeeded in coagulating the choroid plexus of a hydrocephalic child using a cystoscope. The first successful ventriculostomy in a baby with hydrocephalus was performed in Massachusetts in 1923. However, it was not until 1970 with the advent of light transmission through flexible fibre optics that neuroendoscopy was reapplied and new and current endoscopic techniques defined.

Neuroendoscopic ventriculostomy is gradually becoming a popular procedure for the treatment of those patients with obstructive hydrocephalus due to aqueductal stenosis, periaqueductal tumour or posterior fossa tumour (Drake and Sainte-Rose, 1995). The rate of shunt dysfunction is around 30%, the infection rate is 5% to 8% per year and neurological deficits are observed in 7% of shunt users (Harris, 1994). Endoscopy therefore presents an attractive alternative in specific patients.

### Preoperative care

There is little difference in the preparation for this procedure, from that required by the child undergoing insertion of a shunt system. Appropriate explanation is necessary and reassurance should be given that this is not a new procedure.

### Intraoperative care

An endoscope is passed into the lateral ventricle, through the foramen into the third ventricle. The floor of the ventricle is then fenestrated and the hole is usually dilated with a balloon catheter. Once all the equipment has been withdrawn, an external ventricular drain may be left *in situ* for a few days, to act as a safety valve should the fenestration prove not to be permanent. Cerebrospinal fluid drained through the fenestration is reabsorbed via the basal cisterns, back into the venous system.

### Postoperative care

The child should be nursed in a head-up position once recovered from anaesthesia, to encourage CSF drainage through the fenestration. This drainage will initially be much slower than that achieved by a shunt and careful observation of the child is necessary including his or her neurological status. Disturbances to the child in the immediate postoperative period, in the form of vomiting and headache, appear less frequently than those in the shunted child, and any symptoms should be treated accordingly. Once again, parental confidence can be enhanced by handling the child under nursing guidance, although care must be taken with regard to the external ventricular drain as previously discussed.

The external drain will be removed after a few days and, presuming that the child has not displayed signs of raised intracranial pressure indicating the need for a shunt, he or she will be discharged home.

### Prognosis

At the university of Arkansas it was reported that patients demonstrated a 50–70% chance of shunt independence and a further 20% showed distinct improvement of symptoms postoperatively following third ventriculostomy and fenestration. The recommendation was that proper patient selection was essential for improved success (Buenolz, 1991).

Features that increase a child's probability of success are as follows:

* obstructive hydrocephalus;
* the child is more than one year old;
* relatively recent onset of obstruction;
* normal ventricular anatomy;
* enlarged ventricles;
* absence of history of subarachnoid haemorrhage or meningitis.

The advantages of ventriculostomy are many, independence from a shunt being the major one. Rapid recovery from the procedure and earlier discharge from hospital are also advantageous for all concerned.

### Discharge planning

The community team involved with this child and family must be adequately informed about the child's treatment and possible future requirements. Wound care and suture removal is similar to that outlined for hydrocephalus. The family should contact the neurosurgical unit if the child does not recover from the presenting symptoms, or should these symptoms reoccur in the future.

## The long-term outlook for children with hydrocephalus

The long-term outcome for children with hydrocephalus is very variable. Although many children with hydrocephalus may appear extrovert and articulate, this may mask an underlying difficulty. Many of these difficulties are hard to assess and easy to miss. A French study (Hoppe-Hirsh et al., 1998) looked at the outcome of 129 children who were shunted under the age of two years and who were followed up for ten years; the final neurological examination showed that 60% of these children had a motor deficit, 25% had a visual or auditory deficit and 30% suffered from epilepsy. Their IQs were variable, with only 60% entering mainstream school and many of these were one to two years behind their age group. Behavioural disorders were frequent and formed a determinant factor for both social and scholastic integration. Hoppe-Hirsh and her colleagues suggest that prenatal screening and counselling should be seen as important preventative measures for this group of families, as well as aggressive medical treatment of the causes known to cause hydrocephalus. They conclude that psychological and educational help has often been insufficient or given too late and that one-third of the children in their study with school difficulties would have benefited from early co-ordinated psychological and educational assistance.

The child's progress and development will be affected by the aetiology of the hydrocephalus, the degree of any underlying neurological damage and by complications such as infection. Parents need early encouragement to allow their child to mature and develop to his or her optimum potential. This encouragement can come from any member of the team but will start with the ward nurse, doctor, physiotherapist and play specialist, all of whom can help assess the individual child's needs and use their expertise in guiding the parents. Each child is different and the levels of attainment of skills depend on many factors. In addition, the individual child's overall development and adaptation to the world is greatly influenced by the attitude of his or her parents and the environment (May and Carter, 1995). Consequently, a family that is confident in the care of its child, coupled with a local community that is supportive of the child's needs, will assist the child in reaching its potential. It is the responsibility of the multidisciplinary team to ensure that this is provided.

## Subdural haematoma in the infant

Infantile subdural haematoma is usually seen in infants under two years of age and in most cases results from head trauma. If the trauma is severe, the infant will become acutely ill and possibly suffer seizures or respiratory arrest. In such cases the parents will describe finding the baby floppy and pale, requiring violent shaking in order to restore consciousness or respiration. Many of these babies are the subjects of suspected non-accidental injury (NAI), so the cause of the injury is highly relevant but often difficult to confirm. The incidence of child abuse is estimated at 15 per 1,000 children per year, with 1,000 deaths per year due to abuse; it has been estimated that at least half of all the children hospitalized for physical injury resulting from abuse have sustained injuries to the head and face (Jesse, 1995). At the earliest safe time, a skeletal survey will be performed, and should fractures be present alongside the presence of retinal haemorrhages, the diagnosis of NAI is made. The police and social services should be alerted and a case conference organized to ascertain the long-term placement of the child. The safety of siblings must also be considered and this may sometimes mean placing them in care until the situation is clarified.

The nursing and medical care of these babies is complex. The immediate care is clearly resuscitation and this may also involve partial drainage of the subdural haematoma via the anterior fontanelle. A blood transfusion is often required. Seizures are common and may be difficult to control in the acute period. Vomiting is also common due to raised intracranial pressure. These babies are usually very agitated due to cerebral irritation and oedema, and any physical handling merely increases their agitation. In addition, they may occasionally have been rendered blind due to cerebral trauma, causing them further distress and confusion.

The multidisciplinary team must have a unified approach to this baby and the family. The presence of a very sick, agitated baby, coupled with the feelings aroused by the likely diagnosis of NAI, requires a supportive team. The team must initially stay focused on the care required by the baby, leaving the immediate decisions concerning the social situation to the social worker. The whole team, however, needs to keep the parents informed, and must attempt to remain non-judgemental. Good communication and documentation are essential for all concerned, particularly if access to the baby by the parents is restricted.

Treatment is supportive and involves recognizing and treating the signs and symptoms mentioned above. The physiotherapist will assist and advise with regard to positioning the child, and aim at reducing posturing and spasticity. Splinting may be required in those children with severe neurological damage and spasticity. Long-term neurologically impaired children will need referring to the community physiotherapist at the appropriate time.

The more immediate needs of these children may necessitate regular tapping of the haematoma; should the situation not improve over a few weeks, a subdural peritoneal/pleural shunt will be placed. The postoperative care is similar to that required following a ventricular-peritoneal shunt insertion. Should a subdural-pleural catheter be necessary due to the viscosity of the fluid, pleural effusions can occur, occasionally necessitating pleural aspiration. The subdural shunt is a temporary measure: approximately three months following shunt insertion a CT scan will be performed and, presuming the subdural haematomas have resolved, the shunt will be removed.

The long-term care of these babies depends upon the degree of cerebral injury sustained. Many will have a significant degree of brain damage; some are placed in foster care by social services.

Those involved in caring for these babies require patience, understanding and gentleness. Prevention of such injuries must also be considered and studies are under way to determine the most effective preventive strategies. The multidisciplinary team should be involved in research and education surrounding these issues, but they must also maintain their position as an objective advocate for the child and family.

## Benign intracranial hypertension (BIH)

Also known as pseudotumour cerebri. This rare group of patients exhibits all the signs and symptoms of raised intracranial pressure – headache, papilloedema and a decline in visual acuity being among the commonest symptoms in children with BIH. The ventricles are of normal size but the CSF pressure is raised. Diagnosis is made from a description of the patient's medical history, an ophthalmology assessment, a normal CT scan and a lumbar puncture which demonstrates a raised CSF pressure (Fishman, 1984).

Symptomatic therapy aims at keeping the intracranial pressure in a range that will not threaten vision; this will include drug therapy (usually acetazolomide), regular lumbar punctures to reduce the CSF to half its opening pressure and, as a last resort, the insertion of a lumbar-peritoneal shunt.

### Prognosis

In children, most cases of BIH resolve swiftly without long-term neurological damage and surgery is rarely necessary.

## A family's view

### Mum's view

Stephen was diagnosed with congenital hydrocephalus when he was a few days old. His mother describes how terrified she was of entering the world of hospitals and how she could not pronounce or even spell the word *hydrocephalus*. She felt comforted by being able to sleep next to her son throughout their stay in hospital, and reassured by the manner and confidence with which her many questions were answered by nursing and medical staff.

Stephen was fitted with a ventricular-peritoneal shunt and his recovery was uneventful; his mother's main memories of that time – now 17 years ago – are, first, how small her son was to undergo surgery and, second, how difficult, but comforting, to breastfeed him during those first days following surgery.

On discharge, his mother described the ward as her security blanket, and wished that her house overlooked the hospital! She says how logic and calmness assisted her in coping when her husband returned to work, and how reassuring it was to know that she could telephone the ward for advice at any time. Stephen's shunt did, in fact, block a few weeks following the first insertion, and again his recovery following the shunt revision was straightforward. At this time he was fitted with a multipurpose shunt – one that could be switched on and off.

When he was two years old, Stephen fell and hit his head; he became unconscious rapidly. On returning again to the ward it was found that his shunt had been switched off by the blow to his head; he recovered quickly once it was turned back on again.

Difficulties started when Stephen's parents tried to place him in playschool. They were met with refusals and ignorance. Eventually they found a playschool that accepted Stephen, as long as his mother attended full time with him. On a routine visit to their local hospital, the consultant paediatrician told them that they would never be accepted into a normal school and that Stephen would have special needs. His parents refused to accept this, despite the doctor's words that he had never seen a child with hydrocephalus attend a normal school. They eventually moved house to be close to a school that did accept Stephen into the normal education system, and one that offered small classes, a secure environment and good 'old fashioned' teachers. The only requisite was that his mother supervised him in the playground.

The neurosurgeon had advised against contact head sports for Stephen and so he discovered alternative hobbies such as swimming, sailing and badminton.

When he was eight years old, Stephen developed a severe headache with vomiting. The GP refused to visit, and refused the family an ambulance to the hospital. His parents brought him up in the car – a two-hour journey. His shunt was again revised. His parents were deeply concerned by their GP's lack of knowledge concerning the condition, and about the ignorance of the community as a whole. Consequently they joined their local branch of ASBAH and obtained a medic alert card for Stephen; they then photocopied the information and gave it to his teachers, relatives and so forth. They found the hydrocephalus network newsletter published by ASBAH informative and reassuring.

Stephen went on to pass his eleven plus, and attended the local grammar school where he more recently passed all his GCSEs, four at grade A+, four at grade A, one B and a C grade. He gave a teaching session to his school about hydrocephalus, and was awarded a prize for hard work. Stephen's parents realize how lucky they are with regard to his academic skills, but maintain that the most important aspect is that he has good health, and is a confident and happy individual.

### Stephen's view

> It is hard to describe my own feelings towards my medical condition . . . it is hard to imagine my life without it, I have no doubt that without it, I would be a very different person. I almost enjoy being slightly different, my hobbies are fossil collecting, robotics and electronics; I feel it's a shame when people do exactly what is expected of them by their peer groups.

Stephen feels that the positive attitude of his parents towards his condition has paid a huge contribution to his own attitude; his parents have always been caring and committed and found hobbies and activities that he enjoys and are suited to him.

Stephen stresses the importance of a suitable holiday insurance when travelling abroad, with an English-speaking doctor available. He feels this gives him confidence, particularly if his parents are not with him. He was initially concerned about the effects that flying might have on his shunt system, so his father flew with him the first time.

Stephen plans to take three-and-a-half A levels, and hopes to study ancient history at a university. He feels extremely lucky 'to have been able to achieve so much academically'.

### An additional viewpoint

I have included an additional view in order to highlight some of the issues and feelings around shunt blockage – a major concern for many families:

> A setback with the shunt set her back for quite a while; she often came back at lunch for a rest – the school were very understanding. We were contacted by ASBAH and a lovely field worker came to see us; however we made a private decision not to join, we were determined to make her feel as 'normal' as possible.

The child's view (the same family) is that she 'gets on with life and doesn't really consider her condition unless there's a problem with the shunt'. For 13 years her shunt worked well and then there followed a series of difficulties over about 18 months, with repeated shunt blockages and infections. She describes her feelings during an acute shunt blockage:

> I felt so awful all the time; I was constantly vomiting, with headaches and dizziness; I kept drifting in and out of sleep the whole time; I was unaware of what was happening; I could hear and understand what was being said around me, but I couldn't respond.

She also had a period of low-pressure symptoms and describes weeks at home when she felt dizzy and nauseous, losing her balance and her confidence, and generally feeling very ill.

In addition, she had a period on external ventricular drainage for a CSF infection. She felt unwell throughout the entire time the drain was externalized and really didn't feel 'normal' until the shunt was internalized again.

Since these episodes, she has had no problems with her shunt and continues with the same attitude as her parents. She is aware of potential difficulties, but views herself as 'normal', and expects others to do the same.

# References

Birdsall C, Greif L (1990) How do you manage extraventricular drainage? American Journal of Nursing (November) 47–9.

Buenolz RD (1991).Endoscopic coagulation of choroid plexus using the Wand. Neurosurgery 28(3): 421–7.

Del Bigio MR (1993) Neuropathological changes caused by hydrocephalus. Acta Neuropathology 85: 573–85.

Del Bigio MR, McAllister JP (1999) Hydrocephalus pathology. In Choux M, Di Rocco C, Hockley A, Walker M (eds) Pediatric Neurosurgery. London: Churchill Livingstone, pp. 229–30.

Detwiller PW, Porter RW, Rekate HL (1999) Hydrocephalus – clinical features and management. In Choux M, Di Rocco C, Hockley A, Walker M (eds) Pediatric Neurosurgery. London: Churchill Livingstone, pp. 263–4.

Drake JM (1993) Ventriculostomy for treatment of hydrocephalus. Neurosurgery Clinics of America 4: 657–66.

Drake J, Sainte-Rose C (1995) The Shunt Book. Cambridge MA: Blackwell.

El Shafer IL, El Rough MA (1987) Ventriculojugular shunt against the direction of blood flow. Role of the internal jugular vein as an antisiphonage device. Child's Nervous System 3: 282–4.

Epstein F, Lapras C, Wisoff JH (1988) Slit ventricle syndrome: etiology and treatment. Pediatric Neuroscience 14: 5–10.

Fishman RA (1984) The pathophysiology of pseudotumor cerebri. Archives of Neurology 41: 257–8.

Guin S (1995) CNS practice in neurosurgery. Clinical Nurse Specialist (9 January) (1) 3–7.

Harris LW (1994) Endoscopic techniques in neurosurgery. Microsurgery 15: 5412–16.

Heidelberg P, Morn K (1995) Current concept of hydrocephalus: evolution of new classifications. Child's Nervous System 11: 523–32.

Hoppe-Hirsh E, Laroussinie F, Brunet L, Sainte-Rose C, Renier D, Cinalli G, Zerah M, Pierre-Kahn A (1998) Late outcome of the surgical treatment of hydrocephalus. Child's Nervous System 14: 97–9.

Jesse SA (1995) Physical manifestations of child abuse to the head, face and mouth: a hospital survey. ASDC Journal of Dentistry in Childhood 62: 245–9.

Kirk E, White C, Freeman S (1992) Effects of a nursing education intervention on parents' knowledge of hydrocephalus and shunts. Journal of Neuroscience Nursing (20 April) (2): 99–103.

May L, Carter B (1995) Nursing support and care: meeting the needs of the child and family with altered cerebral function. In Carter B, Dearmun AK (eds) Child Health Care Nursing, Concepts, Theory and Practice. Oxford: Blackwell Science, pp. 388–9.

Morn K (ed.) (1993) Annual Report (1992) by Research Committee on Intractable Hydrocephalus (in Japanese with English abstract/supplement). Tokyo: Japanese Ministry of Health and Welfare, pp. 223–36.

Morn K (1995) Current concept of hydrocephalus: evolution of new classifications. Child's Nervous System 11: 523–32.

Pople IK, Bayston R, Hayward R (1992) Infection of cerebrospinal fluid in infants; a study of etiological factors. Journal of Neurosurgery 77: 29–36.

Stanton M (1987) Patient education: Implications for nursing. Today's OR Nurse 9(6): 16–20.

Terry D, Nisbet K (1991) External ventricular drainage. Journal of Neuroscience Nursing (23 December) (6): 347–55.

# Chapter 3
# Spinal abnormalities in children

## Spina bifida

Spina bifida was recognized 2,000 years ago by Prior Tay; most children born with spina bifida at that time died of infection or hydrocephalus. Today, with antibiotic use and the treatment of hydrocephalus, most children born with spina bifida have a long lifespan. The aim of treatment is to provide an optimum quality of life.

### Spinal cord development

By the 28th day of conception, neural tube closure is completed. The rostral end develops into the brain and the caudal portion becomes the spinal cord. As this development continues, the neural tube is covered by primitive skin, followed by bone and muscle around the spinal cord. In the case of spina bifida, a section of the neural tube fails to develop in the normal fashion and the associated bone and muscle cannot form around the spinal cord.

There are well-recognized geographical, racial and possibly environmental factors associated with spina bifida. Although no definite aetiological factors have been identified as causative factors in the past (Hayward, 1980) many theories are now being suggested. Factors include maternal use of valporic acid, excessive vitamin A and insulin. Folic acid and vitamin B can dramatically reduce the risk of having a child with a neural tube defect when taken at least a month before conception and continued for the first few months of pregnancy.

### Myelomeningocoele

Myelomeningocoele is the single most common congenital malformation of the CNS and still occurs in one in 2,000 live births (Tulipan and Bruner, 1998). It constitutes the most devastating form of spina bifida, involving the ectoderm (skin), mesoderm (muscle and bone) and neuroectoderm (spinal cord). The lesion may be completely open and leaking CSF, or the disorganized neural tissue may be covered thinly with a membrane, which is derived from the arachnoid tissue and merges peripherally with the surrounding skin.

## Meningocoele

This less common abnormality is a sac formed of derivatives of the normal meninges, and the neural tissue is not exposed. Consequently, there is a better outcome in neurological terms for the child.

## Diagnosis

Intrauterine investigations include amniocentesis. This measures the amount of alpha-foetal protein in the amniotic fluid, which is known to be elevated in cases of open spina bifida. Ultrasound is routinely performed on all pregnant women undergoing antenatal care in the western world, and may demonstrate the presence of spina bifida. Improved scanning techniques are providing greater detail of the vertebral spine, although occult forms of spinal dysraphism may not be identified.

## Clinical evaluation

Open spina bifida is visually apparent at birth. A thorough examination of the baby is necessary soon after birth to establish the degree of neurological dysfunction. The degree of leg movement will be assessed in conjunction with the physiotherapist, and any hip dislocation also noted. Bowel and bladder function must also be assessed. The baby will be examined for signs of hydrocephalus, regular head measurements will be taken and a cranial ultrasound performed as necessary. A frank discussion with the parents will involve an explanation of the possible long-term complications for the baby and the whole family. Presuming the degree of dysfunction is not so devastating as to make it necessary to withhold treatment, then the treatment must commence immediately in the hope of avoiding further complications.

The lesion must be protected from drying out and from abrasions by covering it with a moist protective dressing. Early surgical closure is recommended to reduce the risk of infection, to prevent further neurological damage and to assist in early bonding with the mother by making the baby easier to handle and perhaps more aesthetically pleasing.

## Preoperative care

The physical care of these neonates is probably far easier than the psychological care required by the parents, particularly if the diagnosis was unknown antenatally.

The physical care includes routine neonatal needs such as establishing feeding, ensuring warmth (the baby may need to be nursed in a baby therm or an incubator if the back lesion is very large and nursed exposed), and observing bowel and bladder function. The nurse should assist the mother in these early days and can do much to help establish breastfeeding should that be the mother's desire. Preparing the baby for theatre in terms of cleanliness can help the mother feel involved with her baby's care.

The physiotherapist will be involved with the baby from the early days. She or he will provide a muscle chart as a preoperative baseline, and teach and encourage the parents to perform appropriate limb movements and correct positioning of their baby. Assessment of muscle power and of which groups of muscles are working is an important prognostic factor in terms of future mobility, and habilitation and rehabilitation needs. Assessing milestones and development alongside ongoing physiotherapy will be essential in obtaining the optimum potential for the child in terms of movement and in limiting deformities (see Figure 13.1a,b,c,d,e).

The psychological needs of this family will encompass the whole multidisciplinary team, because with each contact with the family, many issues may arise that require immediate discussion. The social worker plays a key role in addressing many issues with the family, anticipating its needs, particularly as the child's requirements become more evident. Assistance with fares to and from the hospital can be arranged for those on income support, and arrangements for childcare for siblings can be helpful in freeing the mother to be with her child in hospital.

Uncertainty surrounding the long-term complications, coupled with the anguish and sadness suffered by parents, will result in many discussions and explanations, requiring an understanding approach from the team. Each member of the multidisciplinary team must have a consistent message for these parents and good communication is essential to ensure this happens. The ward nurse is usually the central person in this communication process, both in the hospital setting and at a later date with the community team.

The aim of surgery is to repair the spinal lesion and, in doing so, to preserve existing neurological function. When discussing surgery with the parents this aim must be thoroughly explored and understood to ensure there are no unrealistic expectations by the family.

Name of Patient:                                    Hospital No:

Date of Assessment:                                 Assessed by:

| LEFT | | MUSCLE ACTION | RIGHT | |
|---|---|---|---|---|
| Range of Movement | Motor Function | | Motor Function | Range of Movement |
| | | Flex neck -C2, 3, 4 | ███ | ███ |
| | | Extend neck -C3, 4 | ███ | ███ |
| | | Rotation neck -C2, 3 | | |
| | | Side flexion neck -C2, 3 | | |
| | | Flex shoulder -C5, 6 | | |
| | | Extend shoulder -C5, 6, 7 | | |
| | | Abduct shoulder -C5 | | |
| | | Adduct shoulder -C6, 7, 8 | | |
| | | Internal rot. shoulder -C6, 7, 8 | | |
| | | External rot. shoulder -C6, 7, 8 | | |
| | | Flex elbow -C5, 6 | | |
| | | Extend elbow -C7, 8 | | |
| | | Pronate forearm -C7, 8 | | |
| | | Supinate forearm -C6 | | |
| | | Flex wrist -C6, 7 | | |
| | | Extend wrist -C6, 7 | | |
| | | Flex fingers -C7, 8 | | |
| | | Extend fingers -C7, 8 | | |
| | | Thumb opposition -C8, T1 | | |
| | | Thumb abduction -C8,T1 | | |
| | | Thumb extension -C8, T1 | | |
| | | Upper abdominals | | |
| | | Lower abdominals | | |
| | | Flex hip -L1, 2, 3 | | |
| | | Extend hip -L5, S1 | | |
| | | Abduct hip -L5, S1 | | |
| | | Adduct hip -L1, 2, 3 | | |
| | | Med. Rotate hip -L1, 2, 3 | | |
| | | Lat. Rotate hip -L5, S1 | | |
| | | Flex knee -L5, S1 | | |
| | | Extend knee -L3, 4 | | |
| | | Dorsiflex foot -L4, 5 | | |
| | | Plantarflex foot -S1, 2 | | |
| | | Invert foot -L4, 5 | | |
| | | Evert foot -L5, S1 | | |
| | | Extend great toe -S2, 3 | | |
| | ███ | Straight leg raise | ███ | |
| | ███ | Popliteal angle | ███ | |

motor function is assessed using the following scale

- 5 = normal strength
- 4 = slight weakness; can tolerate only moderate amount of resistance
- 3 = moderate weakness; full range of movement against gravity only (no resistance)
- 2 = severe weakness; can only move when gravity is eliminated
- 1 = very severe weakness; a weak muscle contraction is palpated, but no visible movement is noted
- 0 = complete paralysis

**Figure 3.1a.** Physiotherapy assessment (by courtesy of Nikki Shack, senior physiotherapist in neuroscience, Hospital for Sick Children, Great Ormond St, London).

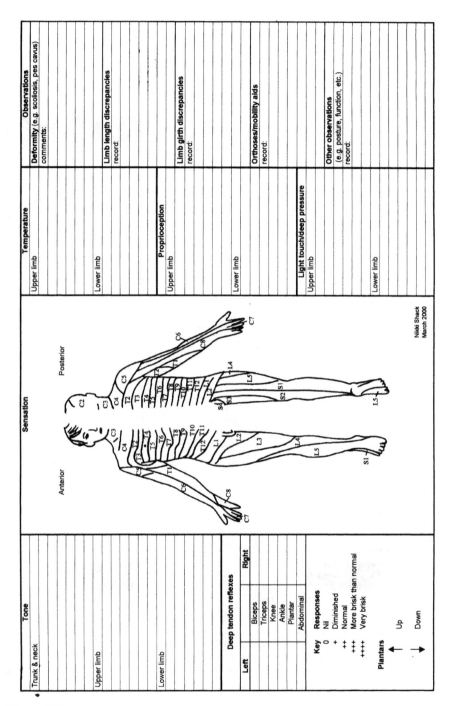

**Figure 3.1b.**

Name:

Hospital Number:

GROSS MOTOR FUNCTION

Bed Mobility:

Lying to sitting:

Sitting balance and saving reactions:

Sitting to standing:

Standing balance and saving reactions

Gait:

Heel–toe gait:

Toe walking:

Heel walking:

Standing on right leg (seconds):

Standing on left leg (seconds):

Hopping – right:

Hopping – left:

Jumping (feet together) forward:

Jumping (feet together) backward:

Jumping (feet together) to right:

Jumping (feet together) to left:

Jumping off object:

Throw / catch ball small (tennis) 2 hands / 1 hand

Throw / catch ball large (football) 2 hands / 1 hand

**Figure 3.1c.**

---

Name:

Hospital Number:

---

<u>FINE MOTOR SKILLS</u>

Drawing:               House

Drawing:               Person

Drawing:               Clock (10.10 am)

Writing:               Name

Writing:               Address

Writing:               Birthdate

Picking up paper clip

Other:

<u>OTHER SKILLS</u>

Cough:

Swallow;

Vision (double vision):

Right / Left Handed

---

Nikki Shack – Senior Physiotherapist – NEUROSCIENCES                          1999

**Figure 3.1d.**

### Proprioception / Vibration

- Upper limbs and lower limbs.
- Use a tuning fork for vibration, otherwise check proprioception by moving a child's limb from one side of body and asking them to on the other side of the body.

### Light Touch / Deep Pressure

- Upper limbs and lower limbs.
- Test light touch using a cotton-wall ball and deep pressure, using finger tip following dermatomal distribution.

### Development / Movement / Posture / Symmetry

- Briefly describe milestones including loss of ability.
  State abilities and inabilities.
- Describe posture of total body in sitting and standing i.e. scoliosis/kyphosis/ kyphoscoliosis in present condition.
- Look for symmetry / asymmetry – if asymmetry is noted document, e.g. girth measurement, limb length asymmetry.
- Associated deformities – note deformities other than spinal deformities, e.g. flat feet, pes cavus, hammer toe, etc.

### Comments

- Note any other significant facts.

**Figure 3.1e.**

## Postoperative care

In addition to the routine postoperative nursing care required by a neonate, involving warmth, feeding and comfort, the baby will require regular neurological observations. The immediate postoperative assessment of limb function will demonstrate if this has changed following surgery. Neurological observations are also important in assessing an increase in intracranial pressure: hydrocephalus may occur immediately following surgery, but is more likely to occur, if at all, in the days and weeks following closure of the spinal lesion. This can cause increased pressure on the back wound and consequently delay wound healing; a close neurological check, head circumference and possible ultrasound or CT scan, will establish the diagnosis of hydrocephalus. Difficulty in feeding, vomiting and drowsiness will also indicate a rise in intracranial pressure, and should be recognized and reported by the nurse. Prompt treatment of hydrocephalus will help to minimize complications and promote optimum recovery and development of the child.

As with much spinal surgery, it is routine practice for the baby to be nursed flat in an attempt to promote wound healing by avoiding any pressure to the wound area. The baby needs to be turned regularly to encourage limb movement and perfusion, and analgesia should be considered prior to any movement. Contamination of the wound with faeces and urine is highly likely and should be attended to promptly to avoid infection. Assessment of bladder and bowel function should be a routine part of the nurse's care: Any dysfunction with micturition may require urethral catheterization, and rectal suppositories may be required to assist defecation. The long-term implications will be discussed later.

Physiotherapy input is essential both at this early stage and in the longer term, to help achieve maximum potential, and to reduce complications. Physiotherapy input will include assessment of sensation, particular attention being given to any disruption in sensation to the buttocks and feet; these 'at risk' areas may cause potential problems in later life with regard to pressure sores, wound healing, seating and footwear. Early liaison with the community physiotherapy team may reduce the difficulties encountered later. Some babies may have associated talipes equinovares and require stretching or splinting. If this is very severe, referral to the orthopaedic surgeons will be necessary.

Once again, involvement of the parents in their baby's care and in any decision making is essential to assist in the bonding process. All members of the multidisciplinary team must share this approach.

The social worker remains an important person for these families in the long term, although this may not seem immediately apparent to the family. In addition to the psychosocial support provided, financial support in the future such as disability living allowance (DLA) can be discussed. The huge changes in lifestyle that these families will encounter will not yet be apparent. However, the skilled social worker will anticipate the potential requirements of the individual family, offering support, advice and practical assistance at the present time and in the future.

**Prognosis**

There is a high mortality for babies with open spina bifida who are untreated. Poor general condition of the baby at birth due to birth injury and hypoxia will result in a poor outlook. Deaths in the first three months are due to infection; later deaths are due to hydrocephalus and renal failure.

For those babies who are actively treated, the prognosis is extremely variable and directly related to the degree of neurological damage. The location and contents of the sac and the degree of hydrocephalus are important factors that influence the outcome of patients with spina bifida

(Date et al., 1993). These findings should provide the parents with realistic expectations with regard to their child's education and expectations.

## Discharge planning

The baby and family will have multiple needs as time progresses. However, the immediate physical needs on discharge from hospital will initially be quite straightforward and will involve the normal discharge plans required for a neonate. Clearly, the GP and midwife/ community nurse will need to be fully informed about the present status of the baby and the probable requirements in the future. A regular assessment by the hospital will provide guidance for the community teams with regard to the baby's requirements.

Physiotherapy needs are long term and a continuous evaluation programme is essential, with good communication between the hospital and community physiotherapy teams. Stretching programmes will help reduce the incidence of contractures and deformities and parents can be taught how to perform these exercises with their child. They can also be taught correct positioning and to be aware of seating positions. As the child grows up, walking training will be required and depending on the degree of disability this may include callipers such as knee–ankle–foot orthosis (KAFOS), ankle–foot–orthosis (AFOS), bracing, and/or wheelchair training. An occupational therapist and social worker will be necessary, particularly in the future as the child's and the family's needs become more apparent.

The family should be encouraged to contact local support groups. The Association of Spina Bifida and Hydrocephalus (ASBAH) has locally based field workers who are very skilled in the complex and long-term care requirements of these families and can offer support and advice.

## Long-term outlook

The difficulties faced by a family caring for an infant or small child with open spina bifida are many and complex. However, all this will seem minimal once faced with the difficulties encountered during schooling, puberty and adolescence. Regular hospital visits to different clinics involved in urological, orthopaedic and neurosurgical procedures will be necessary, and numerous operations will be needed throughout the child's life.

Physiotherapy will be a long-term requirement and the aim of treatment is to establish a pattern of development that is as near to normal as the levels of paraplegia and central nervous system dysfunction allow. Most children will achieve their maximum level of ambulation at around four years of age; a child who is not walking by the age of six is unlikely to walk as an adolescent, and increased walking therapy is unlikely to be effective beyond this age (Mclone and Ito, 1998). For those children who cannot walk, there is a high risk of contractures in hips and feet; for those children who sit most of the time, kyphascoliosis is a possibility. These problems increase the difficulties with seating and positioning thus making wheelchair usage more difficult. Housing may become an issue – accessibility into and around the home and the need for hoists and stair chairs are just a few of the potential requirements. The occupational therapist and social workers will need to anticipate such requirements in advance to enable funding and supply of equipment to occur. A degree of functional independence should be promoted as early as possible, in order to offset overreliance on family and carers during adolescence and adulthood.

In addition to the possibility of educational statementing, the child's own self image will be affected by his illness. There is a recognized 'cocktail party chat' in many children with spina bifida and hydrocephalus, which can make integration into society difficult. Specific learning difficulties coupled with many physical disabilities reduce the likelihood of a good educational outcome. In the longer term, this affects the chances of employment and a degree of independence. A psychologist can assist the child in managing any individual concerns and needs but can also detect the subtle learning disabilities that, if appropriately addressed, could assist the child in reaching his or her maximum potential.

Sexuality can be discussed by parents and the hospital team with the child when appropriate. Children who are reared with a healthy self image and are exposed to normal social situations are more likely to become well-adjusted and happy adults. However, there remains a strong reliance on the family to provide for the many needs of the child, and the severe and long-term social and financial restrictions for the family will influence their everyday lives. One indication of the toll on the family is reflected in the increased divorce rate among the parents of children with spina bifida (Hayward, 1980). The aim of the multidisciplinary team in the hospital and community setting is to ensure that the child has the opportunity to achieve its full potential, while giving the parents the financial, psychological and practical support they need to help them achieve this goal as a family. In addition, the team can assist in encouraging society to accept these individuals in a more positive light, and help them integrate into that society.

## The future

In America, at least 1,500 children with open spina bifida continue to be born each year (Lary and Edmonds, 1996). More than 1,000 women a year in the UK discover they are carrying a baby with a neural tube defect; 150 mothers a year in the UK will continue to give birth to babies with spina bifida and another 850 will go through the trauma of a late termination of pregnancy (Ferriman, 1998).

Prevention of at least 50% of cases of spina bifida is available in the form of dietary folate supplementation (MRC, 1991). Since half of all pregnancies are unplanned, most women do not start taking iron or folic acid supplements until after a positive pregnancy test, by which time it is too late to prevent neural tube defects (Ferriman, 1998). The suggestion that folic acid should routinely be added to flour was made as long ago as 1965 by Professor Richard Smithells, a retired professor of paediatrics at Leeds university; however, the links between supplementary folic acid and pernicious anaemia and, more recently, with cardiovascular disease, continue to prevent this occurrence.

Parents of a child with spina bifida must be encouraged to talk to a geneticist about the risks of further pregnancies producing other affected babies. After conceiving one child with spina bifida, the risk of conceiving another is one in 20; this rises to almost one in eight if two children have already been affected (Hayward, 1980). This applies to babies born with spina bifida or anencephaly.

More recent research indicates that neurological deficit associated with open spina bifida is not entirely caused by the primary defect of neurulation; chronic mechanical injury and amniotic fluid-induced chemical trauma seem to damage the exposed, unprotected foetal neural tissue during gestation. Intrauterine surgery has been performed successfully on a mother carrying a foetus of 23 weeks' gestation with thoracolumbarsacral spina bifida; during surgery, in addition to closure of the spinal wound using skin flaps, a cerebrospinal shunt tubing was inserted and brought out via a skin wound. The baby was delivered at 30 weeks' gestation and the shunt tubing removed. Although long-term follow up is required, at six months of age the baby had reached normal milestones, had no hydrocephalus and had reasonable leg movement (excellent left leg function except for absent plantar flexion of the foot: L5 level; and a right club foot but with right hip and knee extension: L4 level) (Adzick et al., 1998).

Neonates with thoracolumbar spina bifida usually have a degree of developmental delay, hydrocephalus and paraplegia. The above case raises the possibility that intrauterine surgery early in gestation can save neurological function. However, intrauterine surgery does increase the likelihood of a premature birth and this must be taken into account when considering the risks of such an undertaking.

# Spina bifida occulta

There are a small number of congenital abnormalities of the spinal cord not associated with open spina bifida and they come under the heading of spina bifida occulta. Although neurological deficits are often not obvious at birth, the risk of such deficits occurring later in life makes early detection and intervention important. Possible fixation of the spinal cord in an abnormal caudal location can result in the cord suffering stretching, distortion and ischaemia with daily activities, growth and development (Reigal, 1983). The term spina bifida occulta describes the following conditions:

- Diastametomyelia: splitting of the spinal cord by a bony spur or fibrous band.
- Tethering of the spinal roots by a thickened filum terminale ('tethered cord').
- The presence of a lipoma or epidermoid cyst.

The above may occur independently of one another; however, primary spinal cord tethering is found in the different anatomical subtypes of closed spinal dysraphism, most commonly lumbosacral lipomas.

Investigations include a neurological examination, urodynamic assessment and an MRI scan. Most of the deficits are similar to those associated with open spina bifida involving abnormalities of the lower limbs and bladder and bowel dysfunction, but usually in a milder form. A naevus or hairy patch is frequently seen, or a sacral dimple, which provides a valuable pointer to the underlying abnormality. As the child grows, inequality in leg length and foot size may become evident. Spinal lipomas can vary in size but are usually evident at birth.

It is unlikely that surgery will improve any existing neurological deficit and the aim is therefore to prevent further trouble. In addition to repair of the deficit, the aim of surgery is to free the spinal cord, allowing normal mobility of the spinal cord within the spinal canal.

Surgical trauma or postoperative complications may delay recovery, and late tethering may occur due to tissue scarring and adhesions. Furthermore, the natural history of spinal cord disturbance and neurological sequelae may remain uninfluenced by surgery, and lead to inevitable deterioration (Van Calenberg et al., 1999).

Untethering for example, will rarely be able to normalize the neurological situation totally, and deformities can increase even when the motor deficit decreases: orthopaedic symptoms due to muscle imbalance may occur, although pain does usually respond well to spinal cord untethering.

Cornette et al. (1998) suggest that for infants with closed spinal dysraphism and tethered cord, surgery should not be performed prophylactically, but only on the appearance of symptoms. Furthermore, follow up after surgery should be for a long period of time, probably into adulthood.

### Preoperative care

The care requirements are similar to those required by the child under-going surgery for open spina bifida. However, because this group of children may include the older child, psychological care in the form of play therapy or discussion will be necessary to prepare the child for surgery. Suppositories may be necessary to evacuate the bowels as a prophylactic treatment, bed rest and morphine both increasing the likelihood of consti-pation in the postoperative stage. Physiotherapy will include assessment of muscle tone, reflexes, sensation, and power and movement of limbs. Although there are minimal deficits in this group of children, some do have sensation abnormalities that, if increased in the postoperative period, could cause poor healing and skin rubbing from shoes.

### Postoperative care

Specific requirements include analgesia in the form of intravenous morphine as nurse-controlled analgesia (NCA) for the younger child and patient-controlled analgesia (PCA) for the older child. Good analgesia should be achievable; one of the benefits of this is in achieving early physiotherapy, and thus improving movement and early mobility. A period of bed rest will be required in line with local policy before mobilizing, and this can be a difficult period for the younger child. Parents can assist greatly in occupying their child in conjunction with the play specialist, and keeping him or her as immobile as possible during this time.

Urinary catheterization may be necessary, but the risks of infection should be considered and assessed for each individual child.

Long-term follow up will be required for this group of children and their care requirements will be similar to those with open spina bifida, although hopefully some degree of mobility will be preserved.

## Congenital spinal abnormalities and urodynamics

Urodynamic studies are useful both diagnostically and in follow-up studies, particularly for the group of children with tethered cord. Disturbances in the urodynamics of the child often precede clinical manifestations of deterioration and might help decide the benefits of surgery. Urological deficits are unlikely to improve following surgery, the aim being to preserve the existing urological and neurological function. Spinal cord untethering is said, however, to favourably influence the urological function in some patients (Vernet et al., 1996).

Urodynamic studies in the neonatal period are difficult to achieve and best attempted in the quiet, recently fed infant. They are an important assessment as they outline the risk of complications, and suggest the frequency and means of surveillance required in the future. The initial investigation will be a formal ultrasound, between birth and six months of age. Simple urodynamic studies can then be performed, involving a nappy alarm and a post-void ultrasound. Should the bladder function prove normal, an ultrasound and assessment will be performed at six monthly periods. If however, there is residual dribbling of urine, or upper urinary tract changes, a micturating cysto-urethrogram (MCU), cystometrogram (CMG), video and DMSA may be required to more fully evaluate the rest of the urinary tract.

Urodynamic studies and advice can be co-ordinated by a central person and this can be a clinical nurse specialist in urology if available. Intermittent catheterization may be the treatment of choice, particularly in the presence of incomplete bladder emptying and repeated urinary tract infections. Intermittent catheterization requires commitment on the part of one parent or preferably both. Generally speaking, parents cope well and complications directly attributable to catheterization are rare (Joseph et al., 1989). Teaching the parents to catheterize their young child takes patience and encouragement but most parents achieve this skill fairly quickly because it is clearly in the interest of their child. Antibiotic prophylaxis is not routinely used, but reserved for those children with ureteric reflux or repeated infections. An antispasmodic such as oxybutin is beneficial where bladder capacity is impaired due to hyper-reflexia. The child will be taught to self-catheterize once old enough and this gives a sense of control and self-responsibility. However, each child and family must be assessed individually. The child with myelomeningocoele faces such handicaps as reduced mobility, major spinal deformities, obesity and impaired intellect and hand–eye co-ordination. Urinary incontinence may best be managed by using a penile appliance for boys, or an indwelling urethral catheter for girls (Rickwood, 1984). In a few cases, where physical handicaps predominate, construction of a continent, catheterizable, abdominal stoma is appropriate (Mitrofanoff, 1980) but this carries with it the added risk of stenosis or prolapse and should not be considered lightly (Snyder et al., 1983). An occasional role still exists for permanent urinary diversion where these measures prove unsatisfactory.

### Bowel management

Faecal incontinence can pose a huge problem for children with spinal abnormalities, both in management and social terms, and management is a major step towards independence in any child's life. The aim for the child with spina bifida is to achieve a time-trained bowel, rather than true control. The goals of good bowel management are proper stool consistency and the emptying of stool on a regular basis, and at a time that is convenient. These goals can be achieved by a good dietary input with adequate fibre, a good fluid intake and a timed evacuation programme. A clinical nurse specialist in urodynamics is often a resource for the management of these children and can encourage the family to begin a bowel programme as one would normally introduce toilet training to the young child.

Aperients will usually be used, and timed emptying of the lower bowel and rectum will often be managed by administering regular suppositories, enemas or in the more extreme cases, rectal washouts. Formation of a stoma such as an Ace, allows faecal washouts to be performed through part of the colon which is brought out onto the abdominal wall, and is reserved for specific individuals such as adolescents who are acquiring independence.

# Syringomyelia

This is a rare disorder in which a cavity develops in the grey matter of the spinal cord, most commonly in the cervical and upper thoracic regions. The name is derived from 'syrinx', meaning 'tube', and 'myelos', meaning 'spinal cord'. The condition is nearly indistinguishable clinically and radiographically from hydromyelia, which refers to an accumulation of CSF within a dilated spinal cord that contains ependymal lining. Often the two conditions coexist and the term 'hydrosyringomyelia' is used to describe the disorder.

### Communicating syringomyelia

This describes the condition when the cavity or cyst is in communication with the CSF in the ventricles and subarachnoid space. There are various theories on the pathogenesis of syringomyelia, but the end result is a blockage in the exit foramina of the fourth ventricle, resulting in the trapped CSF being forced down the spinal cord (presuming that the communication between the fourth ventricle and the spinal cord is patent). The commonest cause of communicating syringomyelia is Arnold Chiari type 1, in which there is a downward herniation of the cerebellar tonsils.

Pain is a common presenting feature in syringomyelia. Interruption of the spinothalamic tract will cause dissociated sensory loss at the sections affected, and is described as being of a 'cape' or 'mantle' distribution. Muscle wasting and weakness will occur, followed by a spastic paraparesis if the condition continues unchecked. Hydrocephalus may occur and, should the brain stem be affected, syringobulbia, dysarthria, dysphasia, diplopia and nystagmus may also occur.

Early detection of syringomyelia is important in minimizing the long-term complications and consists of history taking, CT scans, X-rays and MRI scans.

## Non-communicating syringomyelia

Spinal cord trauma, tumour or arachnoiditis can result in the formation of a cystic cavity that is not in communication with the remainder of the CSF, and this is known as non-communicating syringomyelia. Treatment is of the cause itself, but the disease process can result in eventual deterioration. The aims of physiotherapy are to assess postural tone and patterns of spasticity, in order to use techniques to reduce or mobilize this tone and allow more normal movements to be utilized. The physiotherapist and occupational therapist will work together and assist in coping with the physical disabilities as they arise; the provision of walking aids and eventually a wheelchair, may become necessary. Although much of the responsibility will once again rest with the family, the multidisciplinary team in the hospital and community setting will need to assess continually, and assist and support the child and the family as new symptoms arise.

## Hydromyelia

Hydromyelia is usually associated with spina bifida in cases of inadequately treated hydrocephalus, or shunt malfunction. The symptoms and treatment for hydromyelia and syringomyelia are similar, so they will be discussed below as one.

## Preoperative care of communicating syringomyelia

A thorough neurological and physiotherapy assessment will provide a baseline for future assessment. Operative therapy is aimed at correcting the causative mechanism. Syrinx to subarachnoid shunt (following tumour removal if present) is the treatment for non-communicating syringomyelia. Decompression craniectomy may be necessary in cases of communicating syringomyelia, and pain can be extreme in the postoperative period. Nurse-controlled analgesia (NCA) or patient-controlled analgesia (PCA) in the form of a morphine pump should be discussed with the parents and, when appropriate, with the child. As with most spinal surgery, the child will be confined to bed for a few days following surgery and a play session involving moving about flat in bed, including turning, can be beneficial in preparing the child for this period of bed rest. The majority of these children are comparatively well prior to surgery and good preparation by the play therapist and nurse in conjunction with the parents may help alleviate some of the trauma in the postoperative period.

### Surgery

Surgery is dictated by the aetiology or by the clinical findings of the individual child. There is not, therefore, one specific operation for treatment of syringomyelia and the care requirements of the child will vary accordingly.

### Postoperative care

A ventricular-peritoneal shunt may be placed if hydrocephalus is present in addition to the other features discussed. However, a decompression operation at the base of the skull along with a cervical laminectomy and attempted decompression of the syrinx is the most likely procedure.

The care required following the latter procedure is similar to that for the child following lumbar laminectomy; difficulty in passing urine or faeces is, however, more likely to be associated with using a bedpan than due to any nerve damage. Analgesia is described in the preoperative section; however, once the child is allowed to sit up and then mobilize, headache can be a persistent problem for many days, thought to be due to low-pressure symptoms. Analgesia should be continued in the form of codeine phosphate, paracetamol and diclofenic once the morphine pump has been discontinued. Physiotherapy should be continued when tolerated and the parents encouraged to assist in this often painful process of recovery.

# Craniovertebral anomalies

The vertebral column, spinal cord, supporting soft tissue and intervertebral discs are all interrelated. Injury to any one of these structures can cause concurrent injury to any one or all of the other structures. The seven cervical vertebrae provide substantial movement of the head and neck, including rotation (made possible by the unique shape of the atlas and the axis), extension and flexion. In children, approximately 70% of all osseous injuries to the cervical spine occur between the first and third vertebrae. The factors that contribute to these injuries include a relatively large head, ligamentous laxity, poorly developed cervical muscles and incompletely developed vertebrae (Crockard and Rogers, 1996). In addition, the cervical spine is not fixed (unlike the thoracic spine, which is fixed to the ribs) and so is rendered even more vulnerable to injury.

## The craniovertebral junction

The craniovertebral junction is a funnel-shaped structure, consisting of the occiput bone posteriorly and the clivus anteriorly; it surrounds the foramen magnum and the atlas and axis vertebrae. The medulla oblongata passes through these bones and their ligaments. The structure of the craniovertebral junction provides mobility at the cost of stability, and in children under the age of eight years muscle development is incomplete. Consequently, there is a higher range of craniocervical mobility, and the effects of trauma are centred around the upper cervical spine in this age group (Menezes, 1993). When these muscles are relaxed or inadequately developed, as in a child under general anaesthesia, the craniocervical region becomes less stable than in the adult.

## Atlanto-axial subluxation

This may occur with or without bone involvement. Subluxation (an incomplete dislocation) can be categorized as follows:

- Anterior. This results from a hyperflexion injury causing rupture of the transverse ligament; the atlas is displaced forward with respect to C2 on lateral X-rays.
- Posterior. This results from hyperextension; the atlas is displaced backwards with respect to C2 on lateral X-rays; it is usually associated with bone fractures, particularly the odontoid.
- Rotational. This results in articular facets interlocking.

## Clinical evaluation

Approximately 55% of the entire rotation of the cervical spine occurs at the atlanto-axial joint; axial rotation is coupled with lateral bending to the opposite side, and the ligaments of the first and second cervical lamina assist in both these movements. If the transverse ligaments are intact, there is rotation, but no antero-posterior subluxation or displacement. If the transverse ligaments are incomplete, there may also be anterior displacement with more potential for neurological injury from cord compression. Posterior displacement is very rare (Fielding and Hawkins, 1977). Despite the fact that the diameter of the spinal canal may be considerably reduced in craniovertebral anomalies in children, injury to the spinal cord in survivors is rare.

There are congenital abnormalities that involve the cervical spine: children with Klippel-Feil syndrome characteristically have an abnormal formation of C1 and C2 with resulting atlanto-axial instability; children with achondroplasia and other related forms of dwarfism have an increased incidence of craniovertebral abnormalities; anterior–posterior atlanto-axial subluxation occurs in 14% to 24% of children with Down syndrome, although the incidence of symptomatic patients is less than 1% (Pueschel and Scola, 1987); ligamentous laxity is also classic in these children.

As previously mentioned, muscle development around the craniovertebral joint is immature in children, and consequently rotatory atlanto-axial subluxation can occur after minor trauma, surgical procedures in the oropharynx (particularly tonsillectomy) and upper respiratory tract infections. If the angular rotation of the neck exceeds 65%, as can occur for example during incorrect positioning of the child during tonsillectomy, complete bilateral C1 and C2 facet subluxation/dislocation with ligamentous rupture may occur (atlanto-axial rotatory subluxation/dislocation). The resulting neck and head position is described as torticollis, and has a characteristic 'cock robin' head position with a lateral head tilt to one side, rotation to the other side and slight flexion; should the situation be long standing, facial flattening and a reduced range of movement will occur (Spetzler and Grahm, 1990). Atlanto-axial rotatory subluxation resolves spontaneously in the majority of children because the joint surfaces remain in contact. However, when spontaneous recovery does not occur conservative measures should be attempted early, involving traction, manipulation and immobilization in a neck collar; complex spinal surgery should only be attempted if this treatment fails.

A complete atlanto-axial dislocation, however, will not resolve spontaneously, and early treatment should be undertaken to reduce the deleterious effects on facial development.

Subluxation can occasionally occur spontaneously (Engelhardt et al., 1995).

### Treatment

Early recognition and treatment of anterior–posterior subluxation is essential (for example in the child with Down syndrome) if neurological deficit is to be minimized or avoided. Surgery will consist of anterior or posterior decompression and fusion.

Early recognition and treatment of dislocation and rotatory subluxation is essential in order for closed reduction (by traction, manipulation or immobilization in a collar) to be successful (Crockard and Rogers, 1996). Although there are differences between rotatory dislocation and rotatory subluxation in the surgical approach to their management, there are similarities in the clinical management of these children: Open reduction will be undertaken only in the case of failed closed reduction, and will entail open exploration of the joint, rather than the more simple spinal manipulation and external bracing.

**Preoperative care**

The need for surgery may be acute, but the majority of children presenting for surgery will have a more chronic presentation. Diagnosis will be made using plain X-rays and CT scanning.

Initial discussions with the parents will usually occur in the outpatient setting. The child and family will be encouraged to visit the ward at this time for several reasons: should a halo vest be required postoperatively, the child will need to be measured at this time to ensure the correct size of halo and jacket are available. During this visit, and depending on the age of the child, this is a good time to introduce the idea of the halo, using dolls in halos if available (these may be donated by the supplier of the halos), photographs and play. The play therapist will assist in preparing the child; should another child currently wearing a halo be present on the ward, clearly this could be a useful source of preparation and education for the family. Preparation does seem to ease the way for these children for what is clearly an unusual and traumatic time following surgery. An information booklet should be available explaining the care required once the child is in a halo. Appropriate clothing should be discussed with the family, provisions being made for clothes that will fit around the halo jacket. During warm months, the sheepskin vest can be hot and irritating and a cotton vest can be fitted underneath it following surgery. During colder months, an appropriate jacket or coat will be required.

Once the child is readmitted for surgery, further play preparation needs to take place along with the usual necessary investigations.

Physiotherapy assessment will be similar to that used for those children with spina bifida. In addition, the child's centre of gravity and body movement will be altered once the halo and jacket are fitted, and warning the child and parents of this possibility may help reduce stress postoperatively. The physiotherapist will teach the child how to roll about in bed, and how to get out of bed by rolling onto his or her front and lowering his or her legs down while holding onto the bed. Such techniques can be taught in a lighthearted manner to help reduce some of the anxieties.

Modern halo systems are light, and are probably as user friendly as they can be. They allow mobilization of the patient, but immobilize the injured parts while healing occurs. However cervical muscle wasting can result and consequently the child should wear a neck collar for a few months following halo removal.

**Surgery**

Realignment by derotation and an attempt at obtaining ligamentous reconstruction by halo immobilization, may be the treatment of choice.

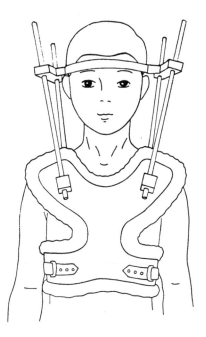

**Figure 3.2.** The halo vest.

Surgery however, may be in the form of surgical fixation, using sublaminar wiring and iliac bone grafting; the posterior approach is the most commonly used, and surgery is successful in 90% of cases (Alday et al., 1996).

### Postoperative care

The usual postoperative care requirements following laminectomy should be implemented. These include regular observation following anaesthesia, assessment of blood loss through the redivac drains and blood/fluid replacement as required, and regular assessment of limb movements. Intravenous fluids will be necessary until the child is tolerating oral fluids, the use of intravenous morphine increasing the likelihood of nausea and vomiting. A neck collar may be used postoperatively and medical instructions regarding the collar and mobility should be noted.

Should a halo be *in situ,* the child will experience fear and distress on finding this, and unable to move his or her head. Mother and child should be reunited at the earliest time that is safe following anaesthesia because the mother is the most likely person to offer comfort to the child. The nurse needs to remember however that the mother will herself be distressed by the situation, and will also need support and reassurance. Relaxation techniques are very useful (for both mother and child) involving deep breathing methods, soothing talk, and a quiet environment.

Adequate doses of intravenous morphine using NCA or PCA should be administered, and a bolus dose given prior to turning the child. Turning should take place regularly; the child is stable within the halo jacket and can be turned safely by placing one's arms around the jacket and the child's skull – the child must never be moved by holding the bars of the halo jacket.

Pillows can be gently pushed between the support bars of the halo jacket and the bed to give the illusion of support and comfort to the child.

Children adapt remarkably easily to life in a halo and once the drains are removed and pain is lessened, they mobilize very quickly with the help of the physiotherapist. Once they are up, it is usually a case of slowing them down! They are initially clumsy in the halo, which seems heavy to the small child. It also adds an extra height and width to the child and this can cause some interesting situations while clambering under tables and other toddler antics! Negotiating stairs can be an anxious time because the child is unable to see the next stair while climbing; the physiotherapist will teach the child to ascend and descend stairs facing the handrail, holding on with both hands and going up or down sideways. For a similar reason, pavement curbs can be difficult to negotiate initially and although the child adapts quickly to the change in his or her centre of gravity, supervision is essential, particularly for the younger child.

Sutures will be removed at seven to 10 days following surgery. It may be necessary to change the sheepskin at this time if soiled from surgery, but this can be quite traumatic and painful for the child and should only be done if hygiene and infection are posing a genuine risk.

## Discharge

Discussion with the GP and district nurse should be undertaken, realizing that they are unlikely to have had any previous experience of a halo system. The hospital should provide an information leaflet to these professionals as well as to the parents to assist with education, and a contact phone number of the ward is also useful. Children being what they are, accidents and bumps will happen, and additional supervision of the child in the halo is clearly required. Should a serious bump occur that dislodges the pins and halo ring, the child will need to be readmitted to hospital immediately and the pins repositioned. The majority of children, however, return to school with relatively few difficulties; in fact they are often the source of fascination and novelty rather than of teasing or bullying. The halo will need checking, and the system tightening at intervals if necessary and this can be performed by the local orthopaedic team if more geographically convenient to the family. The mother will be given a torque wrench on discharge from the neurosurgical unit to take with her for these appointments. The halo pin sites should also be checked at this time and cleaned if necessary. Depending on local policy, the mother may be taught to gently clean the pin sites herself, using saline and cotton wool buds should this be required.

The child will return to the neurosurgical unit for review three months following surgery. Plain X-rays, a CT scan or fluoroscopy (during which the child's neck is gently flexed and extended) will be performed to confirm the position and fusion of the relevant bones. Presuming these are satisfactory, the halo can be removed. This is a traumatic procedure for children, so it is performed under a light general anaesthetic (the CT scan or fluoroscopy can be performed under the same anaesthesia as the halo removal if required). A supportive collar will be applied following removal of the halo system and should be worn during the daytime for a few weeks. Children usually find that a soft collar offers insufficient support following halo removal and a padded hard collar, such as a Philadelphia collar, is therefore preferable.

If appropriate, the child can be discharged home the same day following halo removal. Further surgical treatment should not be required, since both the torticollis and the underlying abnormality should now be corrected.

# A family's view following spinal surgery

Following a normal pregnancy, Sarah was born with a large birthmark on her buttocks and lower back. Her limb function and tone was normal, as were her bowel and bladder functions. Investigations revealed spinal dysraphism, with an angiolipoma, and a large naevus birthmark. The naevus gradually faded spontaneously and routine MRI spinal scans and urodynamic studies were undertaken. When she was two years old, surgery was performed and minimal resection of a large angioma and lipoma undertaken. A year later, Sarah suffered repeated urinary tract infections – she was not co-operative with urodynamic investigations, and was commenced on long-term prophylactic antibiotics.

At age four, Sarah remained fully mobile, but with increasing leg pain and difficulty in micturition. A further MRI scan was performed, surgery was discussed and her parents wished to have time to consider whether the risks associated with further surgery were warranted. Sarah's mother was taught to intermittently catheterize her, urodynamic studies demonstrating that she was not emptying her bladder fully on micturition. Diet was also discussed with the parents, as Sarah tended to be constipated.

Following neurological deterioration, Sarah was booked for spinal surgery.

She was six years old when she underwent a laminoplasty with spinal untethering and excision of a cutaneous sacral lipoma. Surgery was performed by a neurosurgeon and plastic surgeon.

**Mum's view**

> We were shocked when Sarah was born. The birthmark was huge and took ages to fade; her back had a big lump on it. She seemed so normal in every other way, so we just got on with it. There were so many hospital visits, lots of different teams and wards. Her first surgery was easier; she was too young to understand. I could stay with her in hospital, which was wonderful. As she grew up, she used to look at her back in the mirror, we tried to play it down so it didn't become an issue, but she did get teased at school.

Sarah was able to undertake all physical activities, so she could play with her friends as normal. Once she was on antibiotics and intermittent catheterization her life quality improved. However, once she started suffering from leg pain, her parents had to decide on the option of further surgery. There were no guarantees that surgery would be successful, and there was a possibility that she might be harmed from surgery. The decision was difficult, but almost inevitable. Her parents did talk to her about her back, staying in hospital and surgery, and Sarah seemed very accepting. She loved her preoperative day in hospital, but although she was prepared for surgery by both her mother and the ward play specialist, she was quite shocked and upset following surgery.

Mother found the first few days following surgery exhausting and difficult, but once Sarah was more comfortable, she too relaxed. The morphine pump was useful but mum was not convinced that it was sufficient initially, and the pain team was called to review analgesia. Moving in bed was traumatic despite analgesia and Sarah was distressed and miserable for the first day postoperatively. Nausea was controlled with antiemetics. Sarah was catheterized for the period of bed rest, which lasted for a week.

Mum says that Sarah became bored and demanding once she felt better. She herself valued being able to stay with her daughter but describes how difficult it is to occupy your child in bed, for a week. She appreciated the presence of the play specialist who helped occupy Sarah, and the nurses, who in addition to providing care, befriended Sarah and gave her mother a break.

The plastic surgery team wished to look at the wound intermittently during the week, and this was traumatic for Sarah. Entonox was used in an attempt to minimize her distress and discomfort, but compliance was a problem and this technique was consequently abandoned. Mum dreaded the dressing changes, and felt the only way to deal with it was to 'get on with it'. She stayed with Sarah throughout the procedure, which she felt was supportive, but 'awful'.

Mum says she is unsure what the future holds for Sarah, that she hopes all will now be OK for her. It is still early days following surgery and they will 'just have to wait and see'.

### Sarah's view

Sarah told me that she didn't know why she had to have an operation, because there was nothing wrong with her and she wasn't ill. She explained to me that 'Mummy said I had to have it done'. (Her mother said that Sarah worried about how her back looked, and that she had explained to her that the operation would make her back look better.) I asked Sarah if she ever had problems passing urine, or if she had ever been in hospital before, to which she answered 'no!'

Despite preparation prior to theatre from both the play specialist and her mother, Sarah did have misconceptions following her operation. She thought that she was kept in bed (she was on bed rest for a week following surgery) because her legs did not work any more and she wouldn't be able to walk again; that no one was telling her these things, and that they thought she did not know. During her preparation, Sarah asked if she might die, and whether she would be on one of those monitors that she'd seen on television 'when the line went flat and everyone cried'. Following surgery, Sarah's back hurt, once the catheter was removed she had difficulty in passing urine, and she also had difficulty in opening her bowels – this had not happened before her operation, and she again thought that something had gone wrong and that no one was telling her.

Sarah hated having her dressings done. She was also bored. She said she liked having Mummy with her all the time. She was curious about the other children and she liked the nurses (except when they did the dressings). She did not miss school or her friends, and was not worried about getting out of hospital. Once she was allowed off bed rest, she mobilized quickly with the aid of the physiotherapist, but was cross that her legs were 'wobbly and sore'. As the operation was to make her better, why did her legs hurt now, when they didn't hurt before the operation?

Despite being an extrovert little girl, Sarah would not talk to any of the male doctors; we discovered that this was because they never said who they were, and since she did not know their names, she was not going to talk to them! The nurses, however, introduced themselves and explained what they were going to do, so she talked back to them. On future visits, Sarah enjoyed visiting the ward but became wary if anyone wanted to check her back wound, becoming upset and tearful very quickly.

She thought that her back 'looked OK' but she did not want another operation!

## Halo hints

### Hairwashing

This can be difficult. The sheepskin should be prevented from getting wet by placing a towel around the child; if possible, lie or hold the child securely over the edge of the bed, rather than getting the child to bend over a basin. Avoid bumping the pins as this can be painful and could loosen them.

### Pin cleaning

Once the child is fully mobile, the head pins may become sore and encrusted. They may be gently cleaned with saline and cotton wool in accordance with hospital policy. Occasionally, a short course of antibiotics may be necessary; in extreme cases, individual head pins may need to be repositioned under a short anaesthetic.

### Vest care

Should the sheepskin become wet, it should be dried with a hairdryer. Parents must never attempt to dislodge or remove the sheepskin.

### Skin care

The child must not have a shower or a bath, so only accessible areas can be cleaned and dried.

### Stairs

Going up and down stairs can be difficult when you can't see where your feet are going! This applies both to life in the halo, and following its removal, when neck movement will remain severely restricted. The physiotherapist will ensure the child is able to manage stairs prior to discharge, but parents may need to be extra vigilant initially once home.

*Bed*

Getting in and out of bed can take practice when in the halo and following its removal due to the neck movement restriction. The child will find it easier to roll onto one side before attempting to sit upright.

*Balance*

The child will find balance is unstable within the halo and the physiotherapist can help the child adjust to this.

*Muscle weakness*

Following removal of the halo, the neck will be stable but uncomfortable until the muscles have regained some strength. A supportive collar should be worn during the day for four to six weeks.

*Sports*

Sports should be avoided until a discussion with the surgeon has occurred six weeks following removal of the halo. Individual instructions will be given to the family as to the longer term plans, but rough sports such as rugby should clearly be avoided.

*Reading/writing*

The child will have difficulty in reading and writing at a desk and tilting the desk can be helpful.

*Travelling*

The child in a halo should wear a seat belt when in the car.

*Scarring*

Once treatment is complete and the halo removed, scars from the head pins will be evident. Little can be done about this, although clearly a fringe will hide the scars. The use of primrose oil or similar oils known to promote scar improvement, can be beneficial in minimizing residual scarring.

# References

Alday R, Lobato RD, Gomez P (1996) Cervical spine fractures. In Palmer J (ed.) Neurosurgery. London: Churchill Livingstone Inc, pp. 723–36.

Azdick NS, Sutton LN, Crambleholme TM, Flake AW (1998) Successful fetal surgery for spina bifida (letter). Lancet 352: 1675–1676.

Cornette L, Verpoorten C, Lagae L, Van Calenberg F, Vereecken R, Casaer P (1998) Tethered cord syndrome in occult spinal dysraphism. Timing and outcome of surgical release. Neurology 50: 1761–5.

Crockard A, Rogers M (1996) Open reduction of traumatic atlanto axial rotatory dislocation with use of the extreme lateral approach. Journal of Bone and Joint Surgery 78A(3): 431–3.

Date I, Yasurno Y, Asari S, Ohmoto T (1993) Long-term outcome in surgically treated spina bifida cystica. Surgery Neurology 40: 471–5.

Engelhardt P, Frohlich D, Magerl F (1995) Atlanto-axial rotational subluxation in children: therapy in delayed diagnosis. Z Ortho Ihre Grenzgeb 133(3): 196–201.

Ferriman A (1998) Why we need flour power. The Independent (1 December 1998).

Fielding JW, Hawkins RJ (1977) Atlanto-axial rotatory fixation. Journal of Bone and Joint Surgery 59A: 37–44.

Hayward R (1980) The Essentials of Neurosurgery. Oxford: Blackwell Scientific Publications, p. 192.

Joseph DB, Bauer SB, Colodny AH, Mandell J, Retik AB (1989) Clean, intermittent catheterisation of infants with neurogenic bladder. Pediatrics 84: 78–82.

Lary JM, Edmonds LD (1996) Prevalence of spina bifida at birth. United States, 1990–1993. A comparison of two surveillance systems. MMWR CDC Surveillance Summary 45: 15–26.

Mclone D, Ito J (1998) An introduction to spina bifida. Chicago IL: Children's Memorial Spina Bifida Team.

Menezes AH (1993) Normal and abnormal development of the craniocervical junction. In Hoff JT, Crockard A, Hayward R (eds) Neurosurgery – The Scientific Practice of Clinical Practice. 2 edn. London: Blackwell Scientific, pp. 63–83.

Mitrofanoff P (1980) Cystostomie continente transappendiculaire dans le traitment des vessis neurologique. Chirurgie Pediatrique 21: 297–301.

MRC Vitamin Study Research Group (1991) Prevention of neural tube defects. Results of the Medical Research Council vitamin study. Lancet 338: 131–7.

Pueschel SM, Scola F (1987) Atlantoaxial instability in individuals with Down's syndrome: epidemiological, radiographic and clinical studies. Pediatrics 80: 555.

Reigal DH (1983). Tethered spinal cord. In Humphreys MP (ed.) Concepts in Pediatric Neurosurgery 4. Basel: S Karger, pp. 142–64.

Rickwood AMK (1984) Use of internal urethrotomy to reserve upper renal tract dilatation in children with neurogenic bladder dysfunction. British Journal of Urology 54(292): 2–4.

Snyder HM, Kalichman LA, Charney E, Ducket JW (1983) Vesicotomy for neurogenic bladder with spina bifida: follow up. Journal of Urology 130: 924–6.

Spetzler RF, Grahm TW (1990) The far-lateral approach to the inferior clivus and the upper cervical region. Technical note. BNI Quarterly 6: 35–8.

Tulipan N, Bruner J (1992) Myelomeningocoele repair in utero, a report of three cases. Paediatric Neurosurgery 28: 177–80.

Van Calenberg F, Vanvolsem S, Verpoorten C, Lagae L, Casaer P, Plets C (1999) Results after surgery for lumbosacral lipoma: the significance of early and late worsening. Child's Nervous System 15: 439–43.

Vernet O, Farmer JP, Houle A, Montes J (1996) Impact of urodynamic studies on the surgical management of spinal cord untethering. Journal of Neurosurgery 85: 555–9.

# Chapter 4
# Brain tumours

Rickman Godley performed the first successful craniotomy for removal of a brain tumour in 1884, although the patient died of meningitis 10 days later (Ainsworth, 1989). The procedure of craniotomy is believed to be 2,000 years old, when primitive man used this method in an attempt to rid sick tribal members of demons.

Today, craniotomy/craniectomy is used for the removal of brain tumours and surgery still constitutes the primary therapy for tumour eradication. Nowadays, however, it is often just the starting point of treatment, which consists of radiotherapy and chemotherapy in addition to surgical resection.

## Review of literature in relation to current treatment of brain tumours

Paediatric brain tumours are the most common solid tumours found in children and the second most common neoplasm (Shiminski-Maher and Shields, 1995). Paediatric brain tumours account for 20% of all paediatric cancers (Tobias and Hayward, 1989) and the types of tumours and their location differ from those found in the adult population. Historically, paediatric brain tumours have been treated with surgery and/or radiotherapy, but more recently chemotherapy has been utilized, either on its own or more usually in conjunction with the above treatment. Chemotherapy, long thought to be ineffective in the treatment of these tumours, has changed from its previous usage as a palliative treatment to a more actively used and recognized treatment (Ryan and Shiminski-Maher, 1995a). Chemotherapeutic agents and radiotherapy used in the treatment of brain tumours, however, have a neurotoxic effect on the developing brain (Moore, 1995). Influencing factors in the treatment regime today include the child's age, the degree of surgical resection and the histological characteristics of the tumour. The length of survival following the diagnosis of a paediatric brain tumour and the quality of that survival, have been influenced by the recent advances in neurosurgery, anaesthesia, chemotherapy and radiotherapy (Packer et al., 1989). Neuroradiology and, in particular, MRI scanning have been essential aids in these advances. Along with the increased survival time for the child with a brain tumour comes the recognition of significant long-term consequences of the treatment, and these include intellectual and endocrine functions (Johnson, 1995).

## Aetiology of brain tumours

Tumours of the brain comprise about one-fifth of all cancers during child-hood and there has been an increase in their incidence in the last 15 years, of 15%. This response may be due to better diagnostic services rather than any real biological changes. There are 400 to 500 new brain tumours diagnosed in children each year in the United Kingdom, compared with approximately 3000 new cases in the United States; it is therefore important that countries such as the United Kingdom share information, results and research in speciality centres. The only factors that predispose to the development of brain tumours are certain genetic factors, such as neuro-fibromatosis types 1 and 2, tuberous sclerosis and Li-Fraumeni syndrome (Byrne, 1996). Radiation, including exposure *in utero,* is known to increase the risk of tumours. Environmental factors may be important and electromagnetic fields have been the subject of numerous recent studies, following the increased incidence of central nervous system tumours in areas close to high power lines in America (Byrne, 1996). The results of these studies are as yet inconclusive.

## Tumour types

Fifty to 60% of childhood brain tumours originate in the posterior fossa and these include astrocytomas, medulloblastomas and ependymomas; the remaining 40–50% are supratentorial and include optic pathway tumours, hypothalamic tumours, craniopharyngiomas and astrocytomas (Wisoff and Epstein, 1994). Primitive neuroectodermal tumours (PNETs) can occur at any site. The most common childhood tumours are described below.

### Astrocytoma/glioma

This tumour comprises 33% to 40% of all paediatric brain tumours and most originate supratentorially. Signs and symptoms depend on the anatomical position of the tumour and its histological grade: tumours originating in the occiput will result in visual field defects; those in the motor cortex may result in a hemiparesis and seizures; the deep-seated astrocytomas, such as hypothalamic tumours, produce endocrine disturbance.

Approximately 20% of astrocytomas are malignant, and these tumours are currently treated with surgical resection where possible, followed by chemotherapy in children under three years old and radiotherapy for those who are over three.

Oligodendrogliomas are a type of glioma rarely found in children but differ from those that occur in adults in that childhood oligodendrogliomas are usually malignant. These tumours have a vascular bed, predisposing them to spontaneous haemorrhage; they are also prone to seeding throughout the CSF.

Pilocytic (low-grade) astrocytomas comprise the majority of the cerebellar cystic astrocytomas and are also found in the hypothalamus, optic chiasm and brain stem. Those tumours that are totally surgically resectable should result in long-term survival and probable cure for the child; those that are not amenable to total resection, however (and this includes the majority of the brainstem lesions), may require further treatment with low-dose chemotherapy and/or radiotherapy in the expectation that tumour growth will be halted or reduced.

# Medulloblastoma

Medulloblastomas belong to a group of tumours known as PNETs – primitive neuroectodermal tumours. Medulloblastoma is the most common malignant brain tumour in children and accounts for 20% of childhood brain tumours. There is a higher incidence in the first decade than the second decade of life, and there is a well-known male predominance (David et al., 1997). These are posterior fossa lesions, originating in the cerebellum and often involving the fourth ventricle (with resulting hydrocephalus), and the brain stem; dissemination of tumour cells down the spinal column occurs in 25–45% of all children (Geyer et al., 1980). Symptoms include early morning vomiting, ataxia, headaches, potential hydrocephalus, and sometimes visual disturbance.

After surgical resection, craniospinal irradiation has been the treatment of choice, resulting in a 20–60% survival rate over the past two decades (Shiminski-Maher and Shields, 1995). The value of chemotherapy is continually being assessed and several trials are currently in progress, incorporating radiotherapy and chemotherapy.

## Ependymoma

This tumour originates from the ependymal cells of the ventricular lining and usually involves the fourth ventricle; hydrocephalus is therefore common and spinal metastases sometimes occur (less than 10% at diagnosis). Initial treatment is by surgical resection of the cerebral lesion. The grade of an ependymoma has not been proven to be of prognostic significance and a 'watch and wait' policy will occasionally be implemented in a non-metastatic, totally resected tumour. Currently, children under three years old will receive aggressive chemotherapy following surgery; those over three who have had complete surgical resection will receive focal radiotherapy; an incomplete resection will lead to chemotherapy, possible 'second look' surgery, and focal radiotherapy.

## Brainstem tumours

Ten to 15% of all paediatric CNS tumours occur in the brain stem and 80% of these are diffuse intrinsic lesions. Imaging findings are typical and biopsy is not usually necessary. The vast majority are malignant, and the mean survival time following radiotherapy is less than one year (Freeman and Perilongo, 1999).

Symptoms include multiple cranial nerve involvement and, occasionally, hydrocephalus. The development of MRI scanning has allowed for better visualization of the brain stem, and although the majority of brainstem tumours are malignant with a poor outlook, there are a small number that are cystic, focal and operable. Radiation is the main treatment for all brainstem tumours regardless of whether tissue diagnosis is obtained; chemotherapy may also be used.

## Mid-line/supratentorial tumours

The anatomical site of these tumours, plus their histological diagnosis, make the signs and symptoms they exhibit very variable; the treatment given is based on their histology. A large percentage of these tumours are low-grade gliomas and for reasons that are not clear, they often have erratic growth rates. Included are deep-seated tumours, such as craniopharyngiomas, optic pathway, hypothalamic and pineal tumours. Their symptoms include endocrine abnormalities, visual disturbance, cognitive impairment, personality and memory changes. Although most of these tumours are benign, their position makes surgical resection difficult or impossible, and radiotherapy and/or chemotherapy may be the only treatments possible.

Craniopharyngiomas are the most common of these tumours, accounting for 6% to 8% of all childhood brain tumours. They have a characteristic appearance on CT, and 90% are calcified which can be demonstrated by plain X-ray. Craniopharyngiomas arise either from the pituitary stalk or from the tuber cinereum – the floor of the third ventricle – and commonly extend into the hypothalamus. Craniopharyngiomas are difficult to resect and there is usually significant long-term endocrine disturbance due to pituitary involvement; should the hypothalamus be involved, behavioural disturbance, obesity, and learning and memory difficulties may occur. The effects of the tumour and its surgical treatment can result in a child with defective vision, in addition to an altered personality with significant behavioural problems; in some cases, life expectancy may be shortened because of vulnerability to a hypothalamically medicated metabolic crisis. Due to the morbidity associated with radical surgical removal, more conservative methods of treatment are currently being attempted, including cyst aspiration and radiotherapy; intracystic radioactive implants are also occasionally used. An algorithm for the management of childhood craniopharyngioma has been devised by Hayward (1999), dividing patients into those with good and poor risk factors and providing a flow chart for management.

Optic pathway and hypothalamic chiasmic gliomas comprise 5% of paediatric CNS tumours, and occur most frequently in children under five years of age. As many as 70% of optic pathway tumours are associated with neurofibromatosis type 1 (NF1). Although histologically benign, the behaviour of this group of tumours is highly variable and causes significant morbidity, in the form of visual, endocrine and intellectual disabilities. Surgical excision is normally avoided due to tumour invasion along the optic tracts and nerves, although vision will already have been affected to some degree. These tumours are usually low-grade astrocytomas and are treated with chemotherapy; radiotherapy may be given in the older age group (those children over seven years old), although relapse is common.

Supratentorial low-grade astrocytomas may occur outside the optic tracts and are often associated with cyst formation. These cysts are often difficult to resect surgically and are remarkably resilient to treatment by chemotherapy. A catheter with a reservoir may be inserted into the cyst and this reservoir can be aspirated through the overlying burr hole when the child becomes symptomatic. This appears to be an effective form of management although it clearly ties the child to the hospital in terms of location and accessibility.

Pineal gland tumours account for 3% to 8% of childhood tumours. The majority are germinomas and diagnosis is made on radiological and tumour marking assays, thus avoiding the need for a biopsy: On CT and MRI scanning, these tumours are characterized by their strong enhancement with contrast, enhancing metastases throughout the CNS being common. Secreting germ cell tumours excrete a high level of AFP (alphafetoprotein), which is detectable in blood or CSF. B-HCG (the beta subunit of human chorionic gonadotrophin) may be raised in both germinomas and non-germinomas.

The cure rate for small, localized germinomas following treatment with radiotherapy approaches 100%. The prognosis for children with non-germinoma tumours or metastatic disease, treated with radiotherapy and chemotherapy, is less good.

### Choroid plexus tumours

These rare tumours occur most commonly in the first year of life. Histologically most are benign, but approximately 10% show malignant features (carcinomas). Choroid plexus tumours present with symptoms related to hydrocephalus and are highly vascular. Total excision is the optimum therapy, although the carcinoma is more difficult to excise due to its increased vascularity and invasive nature. Radiotherapy and/or chemotherapy will be used for those children with carcinomas.

### Teratomas

These are the most commonly diagnosed hemispheric tumours in children under two years of age. Most occur in the pineal region, the remainder in the suprasellar or intraventricular region. They contain elements from all three germ cells, often including teeth and hair. Teratomas can reach a massive size, making surgical resection difficult.

Complete surgical treatment is curative for benign teratomas. For the rare group of malignant teratomas, survival is unlikely.

## Clinical evaluation

The variations in presentation exhibited by the child with a brain tumour are due to a combination of focal or global neurological deficits, and are dependent on the following factors:

- compression or infiltration of specific cerebral tissue;
- related cerebral oedema;
- development of raised intracranial pressure.

Depending on the type and location of the tumour, one or all of the above symptoms may occur. The diagnosis of a brain tumour is often difficult to establish in a child, because many of the signs and symptoms may mimic those of the more common childhood illnesses. This delay in diagnosis will frequently lead to anger and/or guilt on behalf of the parents, and much reassurance is required to allay the fears that an earlier diagnosis may have led to a better outlook, which in reality is rarely the case.

Signs and symptoms may further vary depending on the age and development of the child, in addition to the size and location of the tumour, although most children will suffer from headaches. Supratentorial cortical tumours are commonly associated with hemiparesis, visual disturbance, seizures and intellectual difficulties.

Supratentorial/mid-line tumours are commonly associated with pituitary disturbance, visual changes and raised intracranial pressure due to hydrocephalus. Posterior fossa tumours are also frequently associated with hydrocephalus and, in addition, with ataxia, vomiting and nystagmus. Brainstem tumours may involve any of the above plus cranial nerve involvement. The child may have been 'generally unwell' and seen the GP on several occasions, prior to a rapid progression of symptoms that will have alerted parents and doctors to the presence of a more serious illness. In addition to the specific signs and symptoms described above, raised intracranial pressure due to cerebral oedema/tumour and/or hydrocephalus will cause a sudden deterioration in the child. This is due to a phenomenon known as the compliance curve, or intracranial pressure–volume curve: initially, an increase in intracranial volume may occur without an increase in ICP (intracranial pressure); however, once the limits of compliance have been reached, the ICP will rise rapidly with small increases in intracranial volume producing significant elevations in ICP. As a result, a seemingly well child may rapidly become critically ill.

### Increased intracranial pressure and hydrocephalus

If any of the three components in the skull (blood, brain and cerebrospinal fluid) vary in volume due to oedema, haemorrhage or hydrocephalus, the intracranial pressure varies. This results in an increase in head circumference in the baby whose skull sutures are not yet fused. In the child with fused sutures the symptoms include headache, vomiting, papilloedema and an altered level of consciousness. Tumour growth can cause a direct volume increase, resulting in raised intracranial pressure, or can cause a block to the normal flow of cerebrospinal fluid, with resulting hydrocephalus. The treatment of increased intracranial pressure due to a cerebral tumour includes the introduction of steroids such as dexamethasone which can produce an improvement within 24 hours of commencement, and removal of the tumour where possible; tumour resection may resolve the hydrocephalus by releasing the local blockage. An external ventricular drain will sometimes be used as a temporary measure to divert CSF, and a ventricular peritoneal shunt inserted at a later date in those children in whom hydrocephalus does not resolve. Occasionally, a third ventriculoscopy may be performed, thus eliminating the need for a shunt.

Hydrocephalus refers to the progressive dilatation of the ventricles due to the production of cerebrospinal fluid (CSF) exceeding its rate of absorption. Thirty to 40% of children with brain tumours will require a permanent shunt for secondary hydrocephalus (Bonner and Seigal, 1988) and consequently the parents and liaison team must have an understanding of the mechanics of shunts and their complications. These complications may include infection, blockage or disconnection; very occasionally, tumour dissemination may occur via the shunt.

The multidisciplinary team is required from the time of the child's admission, although the child will usually have initially been referred to a neurosurgeon. The diagnosis of a brain tumour will be established by CT and MRI scanning: most hospitals have a CT scanner and images can be obtained pre and post contrast administration; this will have provided an initial diagnosis of a tumour; an MRI scan will provide far more detail, and using particular pulse sequences known as T1 and T2, images can be obtained which provide anatomical details and minor changes in the water content of soft tissues. A contrast medium is again used, which will demonstrate vascularity and breakdown of the brain–blood barrier. Older children may tolerate a CT scan without sedation, but many undergoing MRI scanning will require sedation or a general anaesthetic (the latter being preferable in the presence of acutely raised intracranial pressure). The spinal cord is often also scanned, particularly in the presence of a lesion in the posterior fossa, where the likelihood of spinal spread is greatest.

Various medical and nursing teams will need to assess the child. Emergency surgery may be necessary to insert an external ventricular drain, for example in the presence of acute hydrocephalus. However, surgery for removal of the tumour is ideally performed at a controlled time, when investigations are completed and the optimum conditions for surgery are present (not at 3 am unless the child's condition warrants this!). In addition to the neurosurgeon, an endocrine assessment may be relevant, the opinion of a neurologist sought, and a neuropsychologist involved. The oncologist and radiotherapist will be aware of the child, but will not become involved at this stage unless surgery is inappropriate as the initial treatment.

It may not be necessary to involve a clinical nurse specialist or liaison nurse until a definite histological diagnosis has been reached; the ward nurses can keep the parents informed and updated in these early days and liaise with the clinical nurse specialist as appropriate. The anxiety and uncertainty at this early stage of the disease will cause enormous distress and exhaustion to the family and the nurse can assist by listening to their worries, answering their questions where possible and supporting them at this traumatic time. Anxious parents will result in an anxious child; appropriate information needs to be given, including details of procedures and surgery. Hospitalized sick children will often behave in a manner younger than their years and the location and effect of the tumour may add to this; information therefore needs to be appropriate for the child's developmental and emotional state.

## Preoperative care

The child with a newly diagnosed brain tumour, and his or her family, will have been overwhelmed with information and explanations. They will also have met many new people at an exhausting, confusing and very frightening time. It is therefore understandable that explanations need to be repeated and consistent, as the full implication of diagnosis and prognosis is impossible to take in at once. The family needs to be encouraged to take one step at a time. Reassurance must be given where possible and allowances made for perhaps irrational or unpredictable behaviour. Much time is given to the child, but the family (parents, siblings, grandparents, and so forth) also have needs that must be met if the welfare of the child is to be maintained. The shock of diagnosis and the uncertainty of the outcome, coupled with the grief and loss of a healthy child, can be shared with members of the multidisciplinary team, who can then guide the family through the next few hours and then days, providing support through surgery, the postoperative period and the days anxiously awaiting histology results. A unique relationship often forms at this time between the family and a specific nurse, and can be of invaluable assistance to the family, both in the immediate and longer term aspects.

In addition to MRI and/or CT scanning, investigations are minimal: a blood profile and cross match will be required; a physiotherapy evaluation may be appropriate, depending on the location of the tumour and the status of the child; a thorough baseline assessment of the child should be undertaken by a paediatrician.

Consent for surgery will be taken by the neurosurgeon, who will explain the procedure to the parents and discuss the aims of surgery along with the potential complications. The presence of a nurse during this discussion provides the parents with another source of information, as they often need to discuss specific points the surgeon has made, at a later date. Details such as the timing and length of surgery, the location of the child following surgery (the intensive care or high dependency unit, depending on the individual hospital), the monitoring equipment used and the expected status of the child following surgery can all be answered at a time appropriate for the parents. Thorough preparation is advantageous, although little will prepare them adequately for the shock of seeing their own child postoperatively.

## Play therapy

A play specialist is often the best person to discuss anxieties with a child and play is an excellent medium through which children can display their fears (Belson, 1987). The provision of play therapy is one of the top priorities in providing for a sick child's recovery and wellbeing (Brimblecome, 1980). Preparation for surgery is essential and should be performed whenever possible as it reduces some of the child's fears, and prepares the child for the postoperative period; children cope better with the anticipated, however brief the explanation may have been. They have huge fears of the unknown and many of these fears are based on fantasy, which can often be alleviated once discovered.

Preparation ideally begins by discovering what the child perceives the illness to be and what he or she thinks is going to happen. From this point, the play specialist can explain in a way that the child understands, what the operation involves: for the toddler, this may include use of a doll to demonstrate what a head bandage or an intravenous infusion looks like, and for the older child, preparation may include looking at appropriate books or photographs. All preparation must be assessed on the individual's needs and questions should be encouraged and answered as fully and honestly as is appropriate. Hair shaving is now minimal and always performed when the child is anaesthetized, but the psychological implications of head shaving should not be underestimated in the child, particularly for girls. All investigations, including blood tests, should be performed away from the bedside if the child's condition allows, so that the child's bed is, initially at least, a 'safe' area.

Preparation should be undertaken with the consent of the child's parents and in conjunction with them. They have a unique understanding of their child and this should be used for the benefit of the child.

Play also provides an emotional outlet for the child and enhances his or her coping mechanisms (Harvey, 1980). The multidisciplinary team sees it as a vital contribution to the child's recovery because it promotes normal development in both sickness and health, and provides a comforting sense of normality that helps the child adjust to a strange environment. Although the value of play therapy has not yet been demonstrated by research studies, the reduction of stress in patients, parents, doctors and nurses is being recognized when a play therapy programme has been established (Harvey, 1980).

Once the parents have accompanied the child to the anaesthetic room, their long and anxious wait begins, and encouraging them to go off the ward for a while can be beneficial. A pager is a useful way to maintain contact between parents and the ward during this time, should any contact be required. This time away from the ward can be seen purely as a distraction technique for the family, but it also alleviates the anxiety about every incoming phone call to the ward, which is often incorrectly interpreted by anxious parents as a message from theatre concerning their child.

## Intraoperative care

During anaesthesia, controlled ventilation provides optimum operating conditions for performing craniotomy/craniectomy, by reducing intracranial pressure. There is no ideal anaesthetic agent for neurosurgery because all the drugs presently available have side effects or may cause unpredictable problems (Hickey, 1992). Considerations include the effect that drugs have on cerebral metabolism, cerebral blood flow, intracranial pressure and vasomotor tone. Other intraoperative concerns include the introduction of controlled hypothermia (thus decreasing cellular metabolism and the need for oxygen), and hypervenous air embolus (a potential problem associated with the sitting position frequently used for posterior fossa surgery). Surgery may take several hours and it is the responsibility of the theatre nurse, in addition to the anaesthetist, to ensure correct positioning of the child both to allow access for surgery and to ensure the patient's protection; this includes positioning of the limbs, protection of the eyes by closing and covering them, and the usual attention to theatre protocol, such as the use of diathermy. The theatre nurse needs to be familiar with the constantly new and updated neurosurgical equipment such as microscopes, stereotactic frames, neuroendoscopes, the cavitron, and computerized tumour-localizing equipment such as the Wand. Correct assembly, cleaning and maintenance of this equipment is essential and involves appropriate training.

The anaesthetist and the neurosurgeon work closely during surgery. Any sudden haemorrhaging must be supported by the anaesthetist by prompt and appropriate replacement of blood/blood derivatives. An increase in intracranial pressure must be treated by hyperventilation or the administration of appropriate drugs such as mannitol. Any interference with the vital areas of the brain stem will produce an immediate irregularity or abnormality to the child's pulse and blood pressure, and the anaesthetist will report this reaction at once to the surgeon, who can then choose to stop or proceed with caution. Should the child's condition deteriorate, the anaesthetist will advise the neurosurgeon while attempting to stabilize the child's condition. The theatre nurse can alert the ward nurse as to any difficulties that might have arisen during surgery, although a detailed description should also be given by the anaesthetist. Analgesia should be given prior to the child's return to the ward and, if appropriate, the theatre/recovery nurse can clean any excessive blood/betadine off the child, in an attempt to lessen the shock to the parents when they first see their child.

## Postoperative management

Postoperative management is a continuous process that commences as surgery finishes and continues until the time of discharge from hospital.

Immediately following surgery, the child will be taken to the recovery room, the intensive care unit or the high-dependency paediatric neurosurgical ward, depending on the child's condition, the individual hospital's organized layout, and the medical and nursing expertise available.

The objectives of immediate postoperative nursing management in addition to the routine care of airway management and haemodynamic state, are:

- regular neurological assessment and early recognition of raised intracranial pressure;
- recognition and control of factors that could result in a rise of intracranial pressure;
- recognition of potential complications and administration of the required intervention;
- safety of the child;
- administration of regular analgesia;
- comfort and support to both the child and family.

The specialist knowledge of the paediatric neurosurgical nurse will be invaluable in the accurate assessment of the child and the detection of any complications. Teamwork is essential and good communication and a combined approach from the multidisciplinary team will maximize the child's recovery.

Raised intracranial pressure may occur due to cerebral oedema, haemorrhage or progressive hydrocephalus; this will present as increased drowsiness with a decreased coma score, agitation, increased pain and persistent vomiting. Parents may need to be told of the importance of regularly assessing the child's neurological state, as they may become agitated when their child is disturbed for this purpose. An urgent CT scan may be necessary should the child exhibit unexpected symptoms, and appropriate treatment given. This may involve surgical evacuation of a haematoma, or insertion of an external ventricular drain should hydrocephalus be present. Bradycardia and hypertension are indicative of raised intracranial pressure but are a relatively late sign in young children; sluggish pupils and a drowsy child should alert the nurse to the presence of raised intracranial pressure.

Respiratory depression may occur, particularly following posterior fossa surgery (the respiratory centre is located in this region); blood gas tests should be performed to determine respiratory status and the child supported accordingly. The presence of an arterial line will allow regular blood sampling in addition to providing a blood pressure reading, although in the young child this increases the need for constant surveillance to ensure the child does not pull the line out. Correct positioning of the patient, adequate analgesia and physiotherapy management are all important contributions to respiratory status.

Cardiovascular instability and arrhythmias may occur, more frequently associated with surgery to the posterior fossa and the location of the vasomotor centre. Cardiac function, including the recording of blood pressure and heart rate and rhythm, is assessed regularly: tumour invasion of the brain stem coupled with the effects of anaesthesia may cause temporary and usually insignificant arrhythmias.

Pain following craniotomy is often thought to be minimal. However, pain can result from stretching of the dura, the blood vessels and the falx, and from cutting through the strong muscles of the neck during posterior fossa surgery. The use of a pain tool gives a consistent assessment, and a paediatric nurse should be able to assess the child before pain becomes severe. Rectal suppositories are preferable to intramuscular injections for the majority of children but this can be discussed with the older child prior to surgery. Oral analgesia can be administered once the child has recovered from anaesthesia, is not vomiting, and is not at risk from a compromised gag reflex. Constipation is a common side effect from the opiate drugs such as codeine phosphate, and should be anticipated and treated with regular laxatives.

Hydration is initially maintained via intravenous fluids and electrolyte imbalance is common: in addition to monitoring serum electrolytes, urine output must be measured and any disturbance such as diabetes insipidus should be noted and treated. A small child can pass large volumes of dilute urine following surgery to the pituitary, and a fluid replacement protocol must be in place and instigated immediately. Oral fluids can be introduced when appropriate; babies and toddlers are often soothed by a bottle and each child must be assessed individually. Following surgery to the posterior fossa it is customary to delay oral feeding for 12 to 24 hours; this is due to the possibility of temporary oedema involving the IXth and Xth cranial nerves and the resulting compromised swallowing reflex. Potential aspiration pneumonia is a serious complication and oral fluids should not be given until it is clear the child can maintain his or her own airway.

If seizures occur, they can be localized or general; they can manifest as a presenting symptom or occur as a complication of surgery. Clinical features of these seizures are related to the area of the brain involved; thus a localized abnormal area will give rise to a simple partial seizure with no effect on the level of consciousness; a complex partial seizure will involve both cerebral hemispheres and cause impaired consciousness. Seizure activity increases the metabolic rate of the brain and hence the oxygen requirements. The usual care requirements for the child include mainte-nance of a clear airway, an adequate oxygen supply (an oxygen saturation monitor should be used to gauge this and oxygen administered as neces-sary) and safety of the child from self harm. Rectal diazemuls or paralde-hyde is the usual preliminary treatment, followed by intravenous diazemuls and then phenytoin if required. Should seizure activity continue, a loading dose of intravenous phenytoin is usually effective, followed by routine therapeutic doses. Occasionally, however, seizures remain uncontrolled and the child requires intubation, ventilation and sedation alongside anticonvulsants until seizure activity is controlled. Seizures can be extremely frightening for children if they are aware, and certainly to their parents and those around them. A calm approach from the multidisciplinary team and prompt explanation and treatment will help the situation. The social stigma associated with epilepsy is well recog-nized (Jacoby, 1993), and the British Epilepsy Association produces many leaflets including *Epilepsy and the Child,* which the parents may find informative at a later stage.

Wound care involves observation of the wound for bleeding, swelling and infection. Head bandages may be applied on children following poste-rior fossa surgery where there is an increased likelihood of swelling and possible formation of a pseudomeningocoele. Head bandages are also useful for children with wound drains *in situ* (for 'anchoring' purposes and to reduce the risk of the child pulling them out), and also to keep the wound clean and free from investigating fingers! Each child must be assessed and treated as an individual; head bandages may cause much distress to the child, who may fare better once the irritation of a head bandage is removed and the distraction forgotten. Wound drains, if present, should be regularly measured and the child's haemodynamic state kept stable. Rapid replace-ment of blood/albumin/gelofusin must be given as required. A small child will not show a significant tachycardia or drop in blood pressure until approximately 25% of their circulating volume has been lost: the circulating blood volume in a neonate is 85 to 90 ml/kg and in an infant 75 to 80 ml/kg. Hazinski (1992) recommends that blood replacement should be considered if acute blood loss totals 5% to 10% of the child's total circulating blood volume. Thus for a 5 kg baby, blood replacement would be necessary after a blood loss of 22 to 45 ml, which includes any wound seepage in addition to any loss through one or more drains. In today's current climate however, gelofusin is often given instead of blood when medically appropriate, due to the lack of blood available for transfusion and the complications associated with blood donation and transfusion. The drains will be removed 24 to 48 hours following surgery, or once drainage is minimal; explanation to the child where appropriate, and analgesia prior to removal of the drains, will help minimize the trauma to the child.

Vomiting, which may have been among the presenting symptoms, can continue into the postoperative and recovery stage. Tumour invasion and surgical intervention involving the floor of the fourth ventricle, can result in persistent vomiting. Antiemetics should be given frequently and the child's hydration and nutritional status regularly assessed; while intravenous fluids will address the short-term needs of the postoperative child, the child may have presented to the unit as malnourished and underweight. The dietician should be involved at an early stage and high calorie feeds introduced if tolerated. Parenteral nutrition may occasionally be necessary, particularly in the malnourished baby who is likely to be going on to receive high-dose chemotherapy. Feeding can also become a psychological issue for children, who quickly learn how to manipulate situations and control their parents: the more parents become stressed about eating, the less likely the child is to eat for them. It may be necessary to set up a feeding programme in conjunction with the psychologist. In extreme cases, a gastrostomy or percutaneous endoscopic gastrostomy (PEG) has been used – once again, mainly in cases of young children requiring extensive chemotherapy.

Gastric irritation and bleeding can occur due to persistent vomiting, and also due to the use of intravenous steroids. Medication to relieve this can rapidly reduce discomfort for the child and should be anticipated by the nurse and promptly treated.

Hyperthermia can occur due to irritation of the hypothalamus, areas surrounding the hypothalamus (such as the third or fourth ventricle) or the presence of blood within the ventricular system. Pyrexia must be determined as neurogenic or infection related, so that treatment such as antibiotics can be commenced if appropriate. Hyperthermia increases blood pressure, cerebral blood flow and cerebral metabolic rate. As cerebral metabolism increases, production of the metabolic by-products (lactic acid and carbon dioxide) increases; these are potent vasodilating agents that contribute to a rise in ICP. It is therefore important to control the child's hyperthermia because of this risk of increased ICP. Antipyretic drugs can be administered rectally, orally or via a feeding tube. In addition to medication, control of the environment where possible, and tepid sponging, should be instigated. The lowering of body temperature should be achieved gradually: shivering will further increase the temperature.

Visual disturbance can be difficult to determine in the young, non-verbal child. Prior to assessment by an ophthalmologist, the parents and nurses may notice the toddler squinting or having difficulty seeing toys, which indicates a visual disturbance. Diplopia is not uncommon and fortunately is usually temporary – an eye patch may aid the situation but compliance can be a problem! Visual field deficits may occur and are due to surgical trauma or increased ICP; placing toys or books on the side of the bed where the child's vision is intact, will help reduce frustration for the child.

Motor and sensory deficits will relate to the existing problems exhibited by the child prior to surgery, and to the surgical site. Young children adapt remarkably well to changes in mobility, and with the help of the physiotherapist and occupational therapist many will return to a reasonable standard of mobility. A positive attitude and participation from the parents will assist in their child's recovery. Many of the events outlined can, of course, occur after any neurosurgical operation but described below are some of the complications related to specific sites of surgery.

### Infratentorial complications

Some paediatric neurosurgeons operate with the child placed in the sitting position, thus allowing correct anatomical positioning of the brain during surgery. The child will then nursed at a head-up tilt of at least 45 degrees postoperatively.

Good alignment of the head and neck following posterior fossa surgery promotes good venous drainage from the brain but is difficult to achieve in the agitated toddler. Pain from poor neck control and positioning in the postoperative period can be extreme, and early neck movement and exercises should be encouraged.

Potential cranial nerve dysfunction involving the glossopharyngeal and vagus nerves can result in dysfunctional swallowing, as previously discussed. Very occasionally this is a long-term problem, and a tracheostomy and gastrostomy are required.

Other potential cranial nerve involvement includes the oculomotor, trochlear and abducens nerves, resulting in deficits in extraocular movements. The facial nerves may be involved and also the acoustic nerve. Cerebellar dysfunction is not uncommon following posterior fossa surgery and although in many cases this is temporary, some residual ataxia or loss of fine movement may be permanent.

'Posterior fossa syndrome' or 'mutism' occurs in a small number of children and includes difficulty in verbalizing, mutism, intense irritability

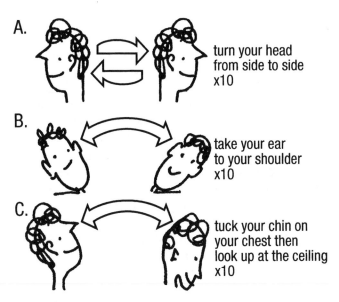

A. turn your head from side to side x10

B. take your ear to your shoulder x10

C. tuck your chin on your chest then look up at the ceiling x10

**Figure 4.1.** Neck exercises following posterior fossa surgery.

and emotional lability, limb weakness and nystagmus (Kirke et al., 1995) among its symptoms. The aetiology of this syndrome is unknown, although it is associated with resection of medulloblastoma, the presence of hydrocephalus, cerebellar insult, resection of a mid-line cerebellar tumour and vascular disturbances. It can last for many weeks or even months, and since it is thought that these children can process information but are unable to communicate orally, their frustration can be understood. Early recognition of the syndrome and appropriate intervention, such as speech therapy and communication tools, are essential. Although the symptoms resolve spontaneously in the majority of cases over a period of weeks, posterior fossa mutism is a stressful complication for these children and all involved with their care.

### Supratentorial complications

Once recovered from anaesthesia the child is nursed at a 30 degree head-up tilt, and ideally with the head and neck in good alignment, thus promoting good venous return from the brain. Correct positioning of those redivac drains not on suction drainage is necessary to prevent a siphoning effect from the drains.

Potential cranial nerve dysfunction may include the optic nerve, the ocular motor nerve, the trochlear and the abducens, resulting in deficits in extraocular movement.

Diabetes insipidus may occur if the hypothalamus has been involved. Seizures and hemiparesis are the other major areas of concern.

Psychological care commenced on admission will be maintained into the postoperative stage. Parents need reassurance and a regular progress update. They value a discussion with the surgeon, who can inform them of the degree of surgical resection and any relevant difficulties encountered during surgery. Nurses can provide repeated explanation to the family, answer questions and provide support. The hospital chaplain, family therapist or social worker can provide more formal support in situations of severe distress; it may also be appropriate for members of the team other than the nurse to provide support to the parents, thus allowing the nurse to concentrate on the care required by the critically sick child.

The extent of surgical resection is best documented by comparing preoperative MRI imaging with an MRI scan performed ideally 12 to 48 hours following surgery. This helps identify residual areas of non-enhancing tumour tissue that may remain in the tumour bed following surgery. The scan is ideally performed soon after surgery, when the child may still be drowsy following anaesthesia. A general anaesthetic may otherwise be required in the agitated toddler, in whom sedation is unlikely to be effective or may be undesirable due to the masking effects of the sedation on the assessment of the child's level of consciousness.

With so many potential complications, the child requires very close observation during the acute postoperative period; emergencies can be sudden and the nurse's observation and clinical skills have a vital role in the child's wellbeing (Ainsworth, 1989). It is also essential that observations are recorded consistently, thus ensuring communication and continuity of care throughout. Children will need constant supervision in the postoperative period, not only because of the potential problems outlined above but also because of the need for ensuring their safety at a time when they may be agitated, ataxic and visually disturbed; in addition, parents are likely to be stressed and may not be functioning in their normally protective role. The task of the paediatric neurosurgical nurse is both challenging and rewarding!

## Long-term concerns

These include:

- the presence of hydrocephalus;
- personality changes (often permanent and caused by surgery to the frontal lobes or the hypothalamus);
- endocrine disturbance (if the pituitary gland is involved);

- cognitive changes;
- change of body image;
- change of family dynamics;
- quality of life;
- long-term prognosis.

Hydrocephalus or shunt malfunction may mimic the signs of a brain tumour including vomiting, headache and drowsiness. A CT scan will be required, necessitating either sedation or general anaesthesia in the uncooperative child. It may be necessary to insert a shunt or to replace a malfunctioning one. Children presenting with pyrexia and neutropaenia (those children currently undergoing chemotherapy) and who have a shunt must have the possibility of a shunt infection assessed. Cerebrospinal fluid is only taken for culture if such infection is strongly indicated, as the risk of introducing infection by sampling is a possibility. In a study of patients with intraventricular reservoirs placed for chemotherapy delivery, 8.2% had positive CSF cultures, although they were clinically asymptomatic (Brown et al., 1987). This raises the discussion of treatment for infection.

The child with a brain tumour presents additional concerns when receiving chemotherapy requiring hyperhydration: the risk of increased intracranial pressure from hyperhydration must be balanced against the risk of chemotherapy side effects due to inadequate hydration. The presence of a ventricular-peritoneal shunt for the treatment of hydro-cephalus might be an asset in the presence of hyperhydration, assisting in reducing raised intracranial pressure. The administration of an antiemetic with a sedative side effect must be balanced against the possibility of the drowsiness caused by shunt malfunction. Both parents and nurses must be encouraged to report subtle changes in the child's behaviour promptly so that appropriate investigations can be instigated if necessary.

Personality changes can be temporary or permanent. Such changes can be caused by surgical trauma to the frontal lobes and pituitary gland, or by the effects of cerebral anoxia. The morbidity associated with radical removal of paediatric craniopharyngioma, for example, has been so extreme with regard to personality changes that surgical technique has now turned to a less invasive surgical approach. If personality changes continue once cerebral oedema has subsided a psychological assessment may be indicated. Personality changes are very disturbing for the family, who will need support and encouragement from all team members.

Cognitive changes following treatment for a brain tumour are well recognized and relate to memory, perception, thought, orientation and abstract reasoning (Hannegan, 1989). Although transient alterations may occur in thought processes due to medication such as dexamethasone, more permanent changes will have severe implications. Changes are difficult to assess in preschool-age children, and an educational psychologist is the most skilled team member in assessing the child and in suggesting management strategies for the child and family. Statementing may be necessary for the child's future education; an initial assessment is made a few weeks following surgery, and then annually. Changes may partially resolve and improve; a study by Phipps (1996) demonstrated that the majority of children following treatment for medulloblastoma showed a decline in their school performance over time, but that the first two years following treatment were a poor indicator of longer term attainment. Repeated absence from school, the effects of hospitalization and the underlying disease in the child with hydrocephalus and a brain tumour, may all contribute to cognitive and psychosocial impairment. The neuro-oncology and liaison nurses can work alongside the community children's nursing services in communicating with the schools about the special needs of these children.

It is generally assumed that changes in body image are felt most by the older/adolescent child. However, loss of hair and a reduced mobility can affect the younger child, who may face bullying and teasing on return to school. Children's and young adolescents' judgements of their own attractiveness are predictive of how they view themselves as people (Harter, 1985). Teenagers have two body images: their own body image and how they think they look, and their ideal body image in the way they would like to look; the distance between the two indicates their level of self esteem (Gross, 1991). Changes in body image are recognizable to everyone and children with such changes need psychological support to help them to adapt. The need for privacy for adolescents in oncology units has been recognized (Thompson, 1990), to enable them to develop their social and sexual relationships. However, although the ideal setting for adolescents in the long term may be an adolescent unit, during the immediate postoperative recovery period, the safest unit will be either an adult or a children's neurosurgical unit, where they will receive the necessary neurosurgical care. During this time, they will have a greater reliance on, and need for, their parents and siblings. Adolescents are at an age where they understand mortality, and will often direct questions to a trusted nurse and spare their parents the pain of their questions. Honesty, where appropriate, is the best approach when answering these questions, remembering to leave a degree of hope and not merely despair.

The entire family is exposed to stress and life changes. The length and complexity of treatment means that one or both parents are regularly away from home, grandparents and neighbours often caring for the siblings. There are work pressures on the wage earner, treatment over a year causing difficulties for even the most understanding of employers. Siblings are exposed to emotional distress and may not receive adequate support as the acute priority lies with the sick child (Carr-Gregg and White, 1987). Problems for the siblings are mainly psychological in nature, with few reported school difficulties. However, jealousy and a constantly sick child in the family can give rise to sibling rivalry and attention-seeking behaviour that the parents can well do without. Early recognition and intervention strategies by professionals will guide the family towards recognizing such problems and hopefully alleviating them.

The implications of complications following treatment for a brain tumour can be profound. The multidisciplinary team, both in hospital and in the community, will be continually involved with the family, working alongside the liaison nurse who can act as a co-ordinator, ensuring good communication and care.

## Adjuvant treatment

Measurement of success in treating childhood CNS tumours must be assessed in terms other than merely survival statistics. The effects of an expanding mass within the developing brain plus the effects of treatment, can have serious long-term consequences for survivors. The sensitivity of the developing brain to injury increases as the age of the patient decreases, thus the infant runs a higher risk of potential brain damage. There is a very fine line between destruction of the tumour and irreversible damage to the CNS in the infant, and treatment strategies must be planned accordingly (Kellie, 1999).

Surgery alone is rarely curative in children with malignant CNS tumours and adjuvant therapy with chemotherapy and/or radiotherapy is necessary. However, as the survival rate improves, so the spectrum of late effects becomes more evident.

Lack of collaboration between centres and countries treating children with CNS tumours, and the fact that CNS tumours in childhood are not common, means that randomized trials are difficult to initiate and complete. To allow biological and clinical research and advances within the field of paediatric neuro-oncology to move forward, co-operation and collaboration between the medical centres involved is essential.

## Radiotherapy

Radiation is used in medical imaging such as X-rays, CT scans and bone scans. In the latter half of the twentieth century, radiotherapy was used to treat neoplasms, sometimes as a sole mode of therapy, and sometimes in conjunction with surgery and chemotherapy. Radiotherapy can be used as a curative, or in palliation to provide symptom relief. When used as a curative treatment, the aim of radiation is to cure the cancer while limiting the harmful effects on healthy tissue.

External beam radiotherapy (teletherapy) is generally used to treat CNS tumours. It can be used to treat the craniospinal axis (the entire brain and spinal cord), the whole brain or as localized radiation. Interstitial radio-therapy or brachytherapy is only occasionally used in paediatrics and involves the implantation of radioisotopes directly into the tumour bed. Fractionated stereotactic radiotherapy is used to treat recurrent gliomas and arteriovenous malformations respectively but is rarely used in children. The 'gamma knife' (stereotactic radiosurgery) provides a large dose of radiation in a single fraction; it aims to cause immediate cell death to the targeted tumour bed; at present, its use is limited in children.

Radiation results in damage to the cell nucleus. If the chromosomal damage is irreparable, cell death is rapid; however, many cells survive the initial onslaught of radiotherapy as the damage does not appear to be excessive, but the delayed effect is fatal and the cell is unable to divide at mitosis (Hilderley, 1992).

Radiation to the brain also causes demyelinization and consequently white matter necrosis, either in localized areas or diffusely throughout the brain. Since most areas of the brain are not fully myelinated until the second year of life (and this process continues until puberty), radiation is withheld or given to the infant brain with extreme caution. Glial cells and the vascular endothelium can also be damaged from radiation, and this can result in oedema and cerebral atrophy (Constine, 1991).

The acute effect of radiotherapy on the CNS includes cerebral oedema in the early part of treatment, which may necessitate a course of dexam-ethasone. Approximately 50% of children receiving radiation to the brain will suffer from somnolence syndrome, which occurs a month or two following treatment; it is characterized by drowsiness, irritability and apathy, is self limiting, and is attributed to transient demyelination. The longer term effects of radiation may not be seen for many years following treatment, or may not be immediately apparent in the young child. Included among the side effects of radiation are cognitive and educational decline, a disturbance in thyroid production, a reduction in growth hormone production and pubertal disturbance. Secondary tumours can also occur, as radiotherapy acts as an immunosuppressor and also a gene mutation initiator. D'Angio and Green (1995) proposed that there is a malignant cell transformation in individuals due to their genetic predispo-sition. Mike (1982) estimated that the risk of a secondary malignancy in the child treated with radiotherapy for a brain tumour was 10 to 20 times the lifetime risk of the general population.

### Palliative radiotherapy

When cancer is no longer amenable to cure, radiation can be used for palliation of specific distressing symptoms and can significantly improve the quality of the child's life. Indications for palliative radiation include pain, and compression of vital structures; spinal metastases are particularly responsive to palliative radiation and can provide the child with a period of pain-free life. The aim of palliative therapy is to achieve palliation of symptoms, and the dose given is therefore the minimal amount required to give symptom relief, thus avoiding the acute side effects of radiotherapy.

### Nursing implications of radiotherapy

The role of the paediatric neurosurgical nurse in preparing the child and family is one of explanation. The radiotherapy department may not be located on the same site, which can cause difficulties for the family; this can be partly alleviated by a visit to the radiotherapy department prior to commencing treatment. The actual radiotherapy will not commence immediately due to the necessity for simulation, or planning; this delay can increase anxieties, and communication and explanation of this process beforehand can be advantageous. Children will need a face mask moulded, to allow accurate planning and reproducible delivery of treatment, and this can be a disturbing experience. Skilled practitioners in the radiotherapy department work with the child in preparing the mask. However, sedation or general anaesthesia may be required on a daily basis throughout radiotherapy treatment in the young child.

# Chemotherapy

Ideally, all children with CNS tumours undergoing chemotherapy, should be cared for at, or certainly linked to, a specialist centre. They should also be entered, where eligible, into international trials where optimum treatment strategies can be better determined. The relatively small number of solid CNS tumours of childhood, means that medical centres must collaborate on their research in an attempt to obtain the best outcome for their patients.

For the majority of paediatric CNS tumours, chemotherapy alone is not curative in intent. However, over the past 30 years, significant advances have been made in the application of chemotherapy and this has now been integrated into the treatment of children with brain tumours. From the 1970s until the early 1990s, chemotherapy was used to delay or avoid the use of cranial radiation. With the introduction of new technologies allowing ever more focused irradiation while sparing the surrounding brain, have come new strategies for those infants with highly malignant tumours. For example, for those infants with a medulloblastoma or PNET and a medium relapse period of just six to 12 months, early use of focal irradiation has been introduced in conjunction to chemotherapy, in an attempt to improve the outcome (Kellie, 1999). The results are as yet unknown.

The blood–brain barrier is a physiological constraint impeding drug delivery to the brain. High-dose chemotherapy can increase the distribution of drugs that fail to cross this barrier at conventional doses, and consequently higher concentrations will be delivered to the tumour (Kalifa et al., 1999). However this process results in severe myelosuppression. Autologous bone marrow transplantation (BMT) and, more recently, peripheral blood stem cell transplantation (PBSCT) have been used to rescue the patient. Autologous BMT involves harvesting cells from the bone marrow of the patient prior to giving intensive myeloblastive chemotherapy. The cells are then returned to the patient following chemotherapy. Peripheral blood stem cell transplantation involves the removal of circulating stem cells (mature blood cell precursors) from the peripheral circulation and subsequently returning them to the patient following high dose chemotherapy. The use of stem cell rescue means that other more drug-specific, dose limiting toxicities occur, including those to the CNS, liver, lung, cardiovascular system and kidneys. However, the advantages of PBSCT over autologous BMT are many, including avoidance of the pain and hospitalization associated with BMT, increased red and white blood cell recovery, a lowered risk of infection and faster reconstitution of immune function (Walker et al., 1994). Peripheral blood stem cell transplantation will remain an area of focus in the future of oncology, and those involved in the child's care need to possess a broad knowledge base of the process, rationale and implications of PBSCT.

There are concerns about the effect of chemotherapy on neurodevelopment, neuroendocrine and growth outcomes of survivors, particularly so for the infant. Other late effects of chemotherapy include hearing loss, renal impairment and infertility. These considerations have influenced the design of curative treatments, particularly in the use of high-dose chemotherapy.

## Nursing implications of chemotherapy

A paediatric neurosurgical nurse is unlikely to also be an expert in administrating chemotherapy. Anyone involved with the preparation, administration, handling and disposal of cytotoxic drugs requires adequate information and training; this extends to anyone involved with the child's care, including doctors, pharmacists and play specialists. People within the chemotherapeutic environment may be unaware of potential risks and are therefore unable to protect themselves; by virtue of their profession, nurses have a duty of care to others and have a responsibility to create and maintain a safe environment (Hooker and Palmer, 1999). Children receiving chemotherapy should therefore ideally be nursed in a dedicated paediatric oncology unit, and this includes the child with a CNS tumour. However, these children may bounce back to the neurosurgical unit during a crisis such as a ventricular peritoneal shunt blockage, or the need for further tumour debulking; should this happen during the child's chemotherapy treatment, the neurosurgical nurse needs to understand such complications as neutropaenia, mucositis and vomiting, and act accordingly.

Following debulking of a tumour that requires chemotherapy, a central venous line such as Hickman line will be necessary, along with various baseline assessments such as audiology and glomerular filtration rate (GFR). This can be a difficult time for parents who, although they may be keen to progress with the next stage of treatment, often face anxieties when leaving the 'safe' and familiar environment of the neurosurgical unit. Communication between nursing staff on both units will help ease the transition for the family; a visit from a nurse or play specialist from the oncology ward with an explanation about Hickman lines for example, can provide the family with a familiar face for the next stage of treatment.

## Outcomes for tumours

### Low-grade gliomas

A total surgical resection of the tumour carries a good prognosis, and may require no further treatment; surveillance MRI scanning is the normal follow up for these children.

For those children with recurrent tumours, such as a craniopharyngioma, radiotherapy and occasionally implantation of radioisotopes to the tumour bed may be undertaken; the results however are poor.

There is evidence that chemotherapy can delay the progress of low-grade gliomas and remove the need for radiotherapy or extensive surgery (Reddy and Packer, 1999). Multiple studies have demonstrated short-term efficacy using low-dose chemotherapy, but long-term outcomes are not yet available. Children most prone to disease progression are those whose tumours cannot be surgically resected, particularly those with diencephalic syndrome.

The optimum timing of chemotherapy for these tumours remains debatable, but should probably be considered for all young children with progressive disease. Long-term follow up is essential in this group of children, to determine the benefits and risks associated with therapy.

## High-grade gliomas

Symptomatic improvement with radiotherapy can give the child and family some quality time, but the expected benefits of radiotherapy must be carefully discussed with the family, as the prognosis remains extremely poor despite radiotherapy.

Chemotherapy given in addition to radiotherapy has made some improvements in the survival of these children (Shiminski-Maher, 1990). The use of low-dose chemotherapy for non brainstem gliomas has been shown to improve survival in some children compared with those who received surgery and radiotherapy alone (Finlay et al., 1995).

However, despite numerous advances and adjuvant chemotherapy, radiotherapy continues to be the most effective therapy for children with high-grade gliomas.

## Brainstem tumours

The prognosis for high-grade brainstem gliomas is dismal. Radiotherapy will provide temporary symptomatic relief – the median time to disease progression is only five to six months following radiotherapy – and the benefits of the treatment must be discussed in an honest fashion with the family.

Consequently, chemotherapy has been introduced in conjunction with radiotherapy, but with disappointing results. The reasons for the inefficacy of chemotherapy on this tumour group is unclear but may include poor distribution of the drugs in the tumour, which may be very large and necrotic. The outcome for children with large diffuse brainstem tumours is so poor that the ethics of giving toxic amounts of chemotherapy with no proven results remain dubious.

For low-grade brainstem gliomas chemotherapy is the optimum treatment, but long-term survival remains rare.

## Medulloblastoma (and PNET)

Historically, radiotherapy has been the treatment of choice following surgical debulking, involving the entire cranial axis. However, survival statistics still remain poor and clinical trials are currently being undertaken to determine the role of radiotherapy and adjuvant chemotherapy following surgical debulking. Packer et al. (1994) state that these recent trials have improved the outcome for some children with medulloblastoma. Combined modality therapy is a prolonged regime, however, which carries financial and social implications for the family, and emotional implications for the child (Hopkins, 1999).

Until recent years, radiotherapy was withheld for those children under three years old due to the devastating effects of radiotherapy on the developing brain, and chemotherapy alone was given. Due to the poor results from this treatment, focal radiotherapy has now been reintroduced in addition to chemotherapy, the results of which are as yet unknown.

### Ependymomas

There is little evidence that chemotherapy is effective on these tumours, despite early encouraging results from the 'baby brain' therapy trials. These trials delay the use of radiotherapy to those children under three years old at diagnosis (due to the adverse effects of radiation on the infant brain), and high-dose chemotherapy is given for a year, following surgical resection of the tumour. Recurrence of the tumour in this age group is not unexpected and treatment will involve a further surgical debulking, followed by radiotherapy.

For those children over three years old, a total surgical debulking followed by radiotherapy offers the best chance of long-term survival.

There has been a modest but gradual increase in survival of children with ependymomas over the past 30 years, but this appears to be due to technical advances in surgery and radiotherapy, rather than the effects of chemotherapy (Bouffet and Foreman, 1999). There is evidence that chemotherapy can induce a partial or complex response in some patients, but there is no proof that chemotherapy can improve long-term survival. Further studies are necessary to develop new strategies aimed at improving survival, with minimum toxicity.

There are numerous rare paediatric tumours of the CNS, and surgical debulking followed by radiotherapy and/or chemotherapy offer the best chance of survival. Co-operation and collaboration between centres is essential if biological and clinical research areas are to be addressed, and if mortality and morbidity are to be reduced.

## Discharge planning

The damaging effect of a brain tumour on the developing brain is of significant importance. Reintegration into society and maintenance of as normal a lifestyle as possible, are two aims of the children's cancer services (SIOP, 1995). Survivors of childhood CNS disease are identified as having special educational needs, requiring physical and psychosocial support after treatment (Glaser et al., 1997). More specific definitions of morbidity must be identified if the requirements of the Children's Act 1989 are to be met and the consequences of cure reduced.

## The neuro-oncology clinical nurse specialist

The care requirements of the child with a brain tumour and his or her family bridge many disciplines including neurosurgery, oncology, radiotherapy, endocrinology, physiotherapy, neuropsychology, speech therapy, play therapy and dietetics. A clinical nurse specialist/other key professional is paramount in co-ordinating the necessary care requirements through multiple treatments, long-term follow up and palliative care. Holt (1993) highlights the importance of communication across disciplines and agencies, providing continuity and communication; it is therefore essential that the family knows which team or individual is co-ordinating care at each stage. The child's discharges from hospital will be numerous and may include (May and Watson, 1999):

- internal transfer from the neurosurgical ward to the oncology ward;
- oncology ward to community, awaiting radiotherapy treatment;
- completion of radiotherapy treatment to community, awaiting chemotherapy treatment;
- discharge to community after each inpatient course of chemotherapy;
- discharge after any emergency admissions due to complications of treatment;
- completion of treatment to community for maintenance care.

At discharge the individual ward will follow its own discharge protocol and the nurse specialist will act as a link to the multidisciplinary team within the hospital and the community. Involvement in the community will include the general practitioner, community nurse, health visitor, social worker, and any other support agencies involved with the family.

The unpredictability of the child's disease is a major difficulty faced by the family. Cohen (1995) outlined commonly occurring events that were found to precipitate parental anxiety. Normal childhood occurrences such as temper tantrums or crying can give rise to anxiety levels that are out of proportion to the situation. Previous misdiagnosis or delay in diagnosis can result in mistrust of specific professionals on whom the family need to rely; guilt about their own delay in recognizing the seriousness of their child's initial illness can be profound and can lead to a lack of confidence in their own parenting skills. There are triggers that lead to anxiety and uncertainty, such as a routine outpatient's appointment, or a change in the treatment therapeutic regime. The family may become familiar with medical jargon routinely used, such as 'survival' or 'remission', but they may not choose to hear these words. Parents express fear of evidence of negative outcomes – propaganda for raising money for example – as this inadvertently raises awareness of the potential disease outcome. New developments in treatment and media coverage increase the parents' sense of desperation. Absence of distraction and relaxation of conscious control, make the night a particularly disturbing time.

Cohen (1995) describes the following: 'Advances in the treatment of childhood diseases have created a population of technology-dependent and medically fragile children whose life expectancy is unknown and whose future quality of life is unpredictable.'

The child and family must learn to manage periods of distress and anxiety, maintain self value and esteem, and to maintain relationships with family and friends. They must therefore be able to access and use available resources for support and guidance, and these should be facilitated by health professionals. An understanding of the family's coping abilities will assist the nursing interventions required for the complex care of these children. Effective listening and communication will help assess factors involving the home situation, body image, re-integration and rehabilitation, family and friend relationships, and coping with functional problems (Barbarin, 1987; Hymovich and Roehnart, 1989).

It is important that the team recognizes its individual limitations and refers the family to a specialist such as a psychologist, psychiatrist or counsellor as appropriate. It is imperative that the family becomes increasingly independent, to enable them to carry on with their own lives, and they require appropriate support and resources to enable this to happen.

## Tumours of the spine and spinal cord

Primary spinal tumours are very uncommon. They can be extradural, intradural extramedullary (inside the dura but outside the spinal cord), or intramedullary. Morbidity associated with spinal tumours depends on the site and extent of the tumour, and the length of symptoms prior to treatment. Mortality depends on the histology of the tumour and the extent of the disease.

Extradural tumours in the paediatric population differ from those found in adults, where 50% of extradural tumours are secondaries. In the child, primary spinal extradural tumours include neuroblastoma, osteogenic sarcoma, Ewing's sarcoma and rhabdosarcoma. Metastases from primary infratentorial brain tumours can protrude into the spinal canal, causing spinal cord compression. Presenting symptoms include localized pain, disturbance to the sphincters and motor impairment.

Intradural extramedullary tumours include meningiomas and nerve sheath tumours, and are extremely rare in children.

Intramedullary tumours account for 4% to 10% of CNS tumours, of which 60% are astrocytomas, 30% are ependymomas and the remaining 10% are teratomas, dermoids and epidermoid cysts (Nadkarni and Rekate, 1999). This group of intramedullary tumours is slowly progressive and the child may have a long history of gradual deterioration. Clinical presentation varies according to the anatomical site of the tumour and can include spinal nerve root compression, local pain and spinal cord compression.

Surgical removal of the tumour may not always be possible (in the case of a very diffuse, extensive tumour) or desirable as the first course of action (as in some cases of infiltrating neuroblastoma where chemotherapy may be equally effective). However, in the face of acute spinal cord compression surgery is usually the primary treatment: loss of limb function for longer than 48 hours prior to surgery offers a poor prognosis with regard to return of that function, although the use of dexamethasone may assist in preserving a degree of function. For those children not presenting with acute cord compression, a transient increase in weakness or sensory loss is common postoperatively; however, only a few patients have a significant permanent increase in neurological deficit following operation (Constantini and Epstein, 1999).

Radiotherapy and occasionally chemotherapy may follow surgery. The prognosis varies according to the extent and histology of the tumour. Drop metastases occurring from primary brain tumours can be treated with radiotherapy but, generally speaking, do not offer a good prognosis.

Spinal deformity remains a major complication of intramedullary spinal cord tumours and their surgical treatment; spinal pain, limitation of spinal movement, torticollis and kyphosis can all occur. Kyphosis is most likely to occur if more than three lamina are removed, or if surgery involves the cervical area of the spine. The outlook is improved if the facets are intact and replaced, but the combination of extensive spinal surgery coupled with radiotherapy on the young child poses a significantly high risk of spinal deformity. Supportive jackets may be required both in the short term, and occasionally in the long term, for the child following laminectomy for tumour – although compliance in wearing the jacket can be an issue in the young child.

A spinal deformity can occur months or even years after surgery, and children should therefore be followed up throughout childhood and adolescence to observe the development or aggravation of spinal deformity.

## Palliative care

Noll et al. (1993) suggest that establishing a rapport and trust with a family are essential in providing support at the time of relapse. A clinical nurse specialist might be the most appropriate person to provide this support; she can also facilitate meetings for the family with relevant professionals to discuss disease progression, the probable effect this will have on the child, second opinions and terminal care. Discussion and reflection will be needed following these meetings.

Good communication and rapport with the community team is essential, as they will become involved if the child is to be nursed at home. Advice regarding symptom control and pain management is often much appreciated: the child dying from a brain tumour is fortunately not a common occurrence, and may be outside the experience of the community team.

Hospices provide an alternative to nursing the child at home or in hospital; they can provide respite during illness, and terminal care in a quiet and informal environment. Those working in the palliative care setting require specific training with regard to giving support and guidance, alongside symptom and medication management. A high staff-to-patient ratio and the availability of family accommodation provide some families with a realistic option with regard to where their child is cared for.

Children who are terminally ill usually know, and although parents often attempt to protect children from the knowledge that they are going to die, such silence can result in unnecessary fear and suffering (Noll et al., 1993). Even very young children can work through their anxieties, with support. A young child, unable to vocalize her own death, drew a picture of a rainbow that went from her bedroom to the sky. On showing the drawing to her mother, the child became relaxed and peaceful.

The aim of the multidisciplinary team, be it in hospital, hospice or in the community, is to provide symptom control and pain management; in addition, the child and family need to be prepared for the child's imminent deterioration and death. Every child and family is unique and their approach to death will vary. During bereavement, it is widely recognized that siblings benefit in the long term from being involved at an early stage (May and Watson, 1999). If they do not deal with their grief in childhood, it may result in complex problems later in life (Black and Judd, 1995). Siblings will take a lead from their parents, gauging their reaction to questions and uncertainties. A four-year-old sibling asked of her mother that if her sister went to the angels (although she didn't want her to) could she please have her bedroom? A straightforward question from a small child, but one that needed an answer!

After bereavement, the clinical nurse specialist should support the family with visits and phone calls for a minimum of a year. A point of contact will always remain, but for the family to move forward it is important that professionals recognize when to withdraw (May and Watson, 1999).

Working with these families can result in the professionals close to them suffering their own emotional pain. While some families feel fortunate to have a professional who cares so deeply for them, others do not want the added burden of other people's distress in addition to dealing with their own. For some families, the presence of hospital staff at the child's funeral is valued but marks the end of that relationship. Each family must be treated and respected as an individual unit, and professionals must have their own support systems in place for dealing with their personal distress. In order to ensure that long-term harmful personal reactions do not occur, and that professionals remain competent in dealing with the next family's individual requirements, strategies for supporting professionals must be in place. This may be in the form of supervision or counselling, depending on the availability of resources.

Families need to know that whatever setting they are in – home, hospital or hospice – they will have skilled, sympathetic help to manage their child's care (Goldman, 1994).

## The future

Many brain tumours remain difficult to cure despite contemporary therapies, and novel treatment approaches are based on an increased scientific understanding of genetics and cellular biology. Although for many childhood cancers such as leukaemia, differential therapies such as immunotherapy (for example cytokines) and immunotoxins are recognized treatment options, CNS tumours remain difficult to treat. Gene-directed therapies may be more useful for these children: if the genetic error can be identified and corrected, the influence of oncogenes can be blocked, loss of tumour-suppressor gene activity reversed or growth-factor receptors inhibited, and the normal regulatory mechanisms can re-exert control (Hooker, 1999). Gene transfer techniques are proving difficult to establish and research continues into this novel practice. Despite the difficulties encountered, the possibility of selective treatment of brain tumours by gene therapy holds great promise (Packer, 1999).

There are many details available for parents regarding treatment options from the Internet. Parents need to discuss such trends with the lead clinician caring for their child, to establish the advantages and disadvantages of the options and the validity of the treatment. In desperation, parents may be tempted to try unorthodox and perhaps inappropriate treatments, where the child might suffer unnecessarily, with no benefit.

Alternative treatments such as homoeopathy are more frequently being used, in conjunction with conventional medical treatments, with some beneficial and minimal apparent adverse effects.

Clinical research trials are an important way forward, offering a prerequisite for advances in treatment. The research nurse is in a unique position, working alongside families, doctors, nurses and trial co-ordinators. The needs and perceptions of these groups may vary and the research nurse can ensure that good working relationships are maintained, with all parties working ethically and efficiently together (Hooker, 1999). Consent to trial participation must be freely given by the parents and without fear of prejudice with regard to their child's care (British Paediatric Association, 1992). Written information should be given in addition to verbal information, regarding the nature of the trial, its benefits, and the alternatives (Hendrick, 1997). Parents may feel encouraged that they are part of a wider treatment plan and trial, and that they are actively involved in research that may benefit their child; consequently they need an honest and frank discussion regarding their expectations to ensure that they are under no misconceptions. The family may feel that should the trial treatment fail, all hope is lost; they need reassurance that participation in research trials does not exclude them from good symptom management and that they will continue to receive supportive care.

Phase one studies are the first trials in humans; the primary aim is to determine the maximum tolerated dose and the dose-limiting toxicities. The first studies are normally undertaken in adults.

Phase two studies examine the potential efficacy of the new drug, the maximum tolerated dose being given and the response monitored. The new drug is then compared with the best standard therapy in which a response was found.

Phase three studies are the multicentred or international randomized trials; large numbers of children are given the new drug, usually in combination with standard therapy, and significant survival benefits determined.

The child with a brain tumour and his or her family must struggle with all the stresses associated with the diagnosis of cancer, and the implications of this diagnosis. In addition to the fears, concerns and hopes, the uncertainty of cure exists alongside the additional issues of neurocognitive and endocrinological sequelae. The loss is therefore twofold: the potential loss of a neurologically healthy child and the permanent threat of the child's death from the tumour. The care of these children and their families crosses many disciplines and is both challenging and rewarding. Ryan and Shaminski-Maher (1995b), describe the following:

> So often, on hearing we work with children who have cancer, and especially children with brain tumours, friends and family members ask 'How can you possibly do that? It must be so hard.' Our response is 'How could we possibly not!'

## Support groups

There are many groups specifically relating to welfare, information, support, wish granters, education and equipment, respite care and holidays. A few are listed on pp. 200–1; but a more extensive list can be obtained from the UK Brain Tumour Resource Directory (see p. 201).

## A family's view

When Simon was four years old, he was diagnosed with a craniopharyngioma. He had a complete surgical removal with minimal morbidity; however he developed hydrocephalus postoperatively and has required several shunt replacements over the past 13 years. He has just taken 10 GCSEs.

## Mum's view

Most of mother's memories have been taken from diaries she has kept over the years.

Following a measles vaccination, Simon changed from being a happy active toddler, to a miserable, clingy, sickly child. He had frequent headaches and was often sick. He was diagnosed as suffering from migraine, and prone to stomach bugs; when it was realized he wasn't seeing properly, he was given glasses for close work and television. When his behaviour became worse, the health visitor told his mother that this was due to jealousy associated with the birth of his brother. His parents knew there was something seriously wrong by this time, 'but no one would listen to us'. They even wrote to a paediatric neurologist at a large hospital – he didn't offer to see Simon, but diagnosed migraine from the description he was given.

It was a locum GP called out by Simon's parents one evening, who finally got them admitted to the local hospital. This GP had worked in a neurosurgical unit during his training and recognized that Simon needed immediate admission. Simon had a skull X-ray performed, which 'showed nothing' and the hospital wished to discharge him that evening. However, Simon had a seizure and his parents adamantly refused to take him home. He was transferred the following day to a paediatric neurosurgical unit, the ward sister telling parents 'that they ought to be prepared to stay for a few days when they got there'.

A CT scan the following day showed a craniopharyngioma. Parents describe their reaction as 'stunned disbelief, coupled with a kind of relief'. Mother wrote the following:

> We were never quite sure if the nurses were trained to give advice and information in a steady trickle, but it seemed to be by far the best way as we struggled to take in and understand a whole new language and a hospital way of life; it was hard to explain to a relatively active four year old that he was seriously ill and almost hard to believe ourselves, since after the initial dose of steroids he seemed brighter for a while. We eventually told Simon that the doctors and nurses were going to make his nasty headaches better.

On reflection, Simon's mother wishes that she had pushed harder and earlier to discover what was wrong with her son; she urges anyone who is concerned about their child to follow their instincts: 'no one knows a child better than his parents'.

During the initial stay in hospital, Simon underwent surgery for removal of his tumour. His mother is grateful that both she and her husband were included in Simon's care and that they were clearly seen as important to Simon's care and recovery. She describes the strain of dividing time between her toddler at home and her son in hospital, how enormous pressure was put on family life, jobs and relationships, how she and her husband communicated on the phone and in writing, exchanging information and updates. She is aware how fortunate they were in that her husband's job remained secure, both in the immediate and long term.

When they were discharged following the initial surgery, mother describes a mixture of relief and concern. She felt terribly alone, with no one to turn to for advice; the GP was reassuring, telling them to contact him as necessary, and gradually they all became familiar and confident with administering Simon's medications (anticonvulsants, steroids and antidiuretic hormone). Simon was apt to vomit for no apparent reason and parents say they 'lurched through those first few months at home'.

Simon was due to start school and the teachers were remarkably understanding, although there were many phone calls in the early days. Simon required a shunt revision shortly after starting school and it took him quite a while to settle down again following this; he was tired and lethargic, often coming home at lunchtime for a sleep. Parents contacted the Association of Spinabifida and Hydrocephalus but felt that they would not join the group as they wished to make Simon feel 'as normal as possible'.

Over the following years, setbacks were mainly shunt related. His mother describes her feelings:

> We have encouraged Simon to feel that he is no different from anyone else, in fact we feel he is very lucky. We have sent him on adventure camps, field trips and even an exchange visit to France, always with our hearts in our mouths, always at the end of a phone, always with the organizers informed and competent. Normally we stick to holidays in the UK, insurance has been difficult. Simon seems to naturally steer clear of competitive sports, but we have encouraged him to try swimming and golf.

Simon was given growth hormone over the years and is now 'a strong, hulking 16 year old, taking life in his stride'. Life is easier with the advent of an oral preparation of antidiuretic hormone, which no longer needs storage in a fridge, giving Simon more independence. His parents have encouraged him to lead as normal a life as possible, hospital visits are now less frequent and life is easier. They feel that Simon sees his initial tumour as very much in the past and only when he has problems with his shunt, does he focus on himself.

Simon's parents found the thoughts that he himself described (below) were revealing, and got them all talking about the future. They feel his success in his GSCEs has given him confidence in himself, and the move to a sixth form college has helped his independence. His household skills are similar to any teenager ('he can cook noodles, and beans on toast'). Communication within the family is good and a mobile phone has ensured that they can always be in contact if necessary.

Simon's parents feel confident that his job prospects are as good as anyone else's, and that they will be proud of him, whatever he achieves. His mother says 'seriously, we worry of course, but Simon really does feel confident and positive, and so do we'.

Simon's care has now been transferred to an adult neurosurgical unit and his parents describe how sad that transition was for them. 'The care we have received has been fantastic, words can't express how grateful we are.' They wish, however, that more literature and information had been available along the way and are pleased to offer their own views in the hope that we, as professionals, will learn from their experience.

**Simon's view**

Simon doesn't remember anything of the initial surgery or time in hospital. He does remember long waits in clinics, blood tests and shunt revisions – particularly how ill he felt when his shunt went wrong and how much it hurt after surgery. Following a shunt revision when he was eight, Simon expresses surprise at how long it took him to feel better. He wanted to go out with his friends, to be free from his problems. 'At this time, I just wished I was someone else, somewhere else, someone with no problems, who was fit and well, someone normal.' When he did go outside, he felt that people stared at his scars and questioned him; he wore a hat, but people still asked him why he wasn't at school, and this increased his feeling of being 'different'. Simon's shunt blocked again two years later, requiring five operations over a period of a month, and half a term off school just as GCSEs were approaching.

This resulted in Simon's awareness of the probability of future surgery, and he is keen to have a ventriculostomy should his shunt block again, so that he may be 'closer to a normal person'.

Simon doesn't dwell on his tumour, preferring to 'get on with life'. He prefers that only his closest friends who understand and accept his problems, know about them. He learned who his true friends were – those who accepted his differences. Taking regular medication has been restricting, but made easier since the advent of oral DDAVP (antidiuretic hormone). A girl once asked him for some of his nasal DDAVP for her cold, and the complexity of explaining to her what it was and why he took it resulted in him trying to keep it out of her sight from then on!

Simon has seen other children with craniopharyngiomas, who have suffered many more problems than he has, and he feels he is lucky to have only a few problems to deal with. He does not want to be bombarded with questions and finds it easier to keep himself to himself when possible. He is desperate to be able to drive and hopes that the damage caused to his eye by the tumour, will not hamper this:

> The tumour has not stopped me from being able to do normal things. I still managed to get 10 GSCEs – 4 Bs, 4Cs a D and an E. I am now in college taking a 3D design course and I'm doing fine. I plan to go to university eventually. I am living a normal life otherwise, and am putting my problems behind me and trying to be a normal person.

# References

Ainsworth H (1989) The nursing care of children undergoing craniotomy. Nursing 3(33): 5–7.

Albright L (1993) Paediatric brain tumours. Clinical Cancer Journal 43(5): 230–2.

Albright L, Wisoff JH, Zeltzer PM, Wisoff JH, Zeltzer PM, Boyett JM, Rorke LB, Stanley P (1996) Effects of medulloblastoma resections on outcome in children: a report from Children's Cancer Group. Neurosurgery 38: 265–71.

Barbarin OA (1987) Psychosocial risks and invulnerability: a review of the theoretical and empirical basis of preventative family-focused services for survivors of childhood cancer. Journal of Pyschosocial Oncology 5(1): 25–41.

Belson P (1987) A plea for play. Nursing Times 1(83): 26.

Black D, Judd D (1995) Give Sorrow Words (2 edn). London: Whurr.

Bonner K, Seigal KR (1988) Pathology, treatment and management of posterior fossa brain tumours in children. Journal of Neuroscience Nursing 20(2): 82–93.

Bouffet E, Foreman N (1999) Chemotherapy for intracranial ependymomas. Child's Nervous System 15: 563–70.

Brimblecombe F (1980) Foreword. In Weller BF (ed.) Helping Sick Children Play. London: Balliere Tindall.

British Paediatric Association (1992) Guidelines for the Ethical conduct of Medical Research Involving Children. London: British Paediatric Association.

Brown MJ, Dinndorf PA, Perek D et al. (1987) Infectious complications of intraventricular reservoirs in cancer patients. Pediatric Infectious Disease 6(2): 182–9.

Brown WD, Tavare CJ, Sobel EL, Gilles FH (1995) Medulloblastoma and Collins' law: a critical review of the concept of a period of risk for tumour recurrence and patient survival. Neurosurgery 36: 691–7.

Byrne J (1996) The Epidemiology of Brain Tumours in Children. Paper presented at the Seventh International Symposium for Pediatric Neuro Oncology. Washington DC: Children's National Medical Center.

Carr-Gregg M, White L (1987) Siblings of paediatric cancer patients: a population at risk. Medical Pediatric Oncology 15: 62–8.

Choux M, Di Rocco C, Hockley A, Walker M (eds) Paediatric Neurosurgery. New York: Churchill Livingstone.

Cohen MH (1995) The triggers of heightened parental uncertainty in chronic, life-threatening childhood illnesses. Qualitative Health Research (February) 60–2.

Constantini S, Epstein F (1999) Pediatric intraspinal tumors. In Choux M, Di Rocco C, Hockley A, Walker M (eds) Pediatric Neurosurgery. New York: Churchill Livingstone, pp. 601–13.

Constine LS (1991) Late effects of radiation therapy. Pediatrician 18(1): 37–48.

D'Angio GL, Green DM (1995) Induced malignancies. In Abeloff MD, Armitage JO, Lichter AS, Niederhuber JE (eds) Clinical Oncology. New York: Churchill Livingstone, pp. 833–49.

David KM, Casey ATH, Hayward RD, Harkness WFJ, Phipps K, Wade AM (1997) Medulloblastoma: is the five-year survival improving? A review of 80 cases from a single institution. Journal of Neurosurgery 86: 13–21.

Finlay JL, Boyett JM, Yates AJ, Wisoff JH, Milstein JM, Geyer JR, Bertolone SJ, McGuire P, Cherlow JM, Tefft M, Turski PA, Wara WM, Edwards M, Sutton LV, Berger MS, Epstein F, Ayes G, Allen JC, Packer RJ (1995) Randomised phase III trial in childhood high grade astrocytoma comparing vincristine, lamustine, and prednisone with the 8-drugs-in-1-day regime. Journal of Clinical Oncology 13: 112–23.

Freeman C, Perilongo G (1999) Chemotherapy for brain stem tumours. Child's Nervous System 15: 545–53.

Geyer R, Levy M, Berger MS et al. (1980) Infants with medulloblastoma: a single institution review of survival. Neurosurgery 29(5): 701–11.

Glaser AW, Abdul Rashid NF, U CL, Walker DA (1997) School behaviour and health status after central nervous system tumours in childhood. British Journal of Cancer 76(5): 643–50.

Goldman A (1994) (ed.) Care of the Dying Child. Oxford: Oxford University Press.

Gross R (1991) Psychology: The Science of Mind and Behaviour. London: Hodder & Stoughton.

Hannegan L (1989) Transient cognitive changes after craniotomy. Journal of Neuroscience Nursing 21(3): 165–70.

Harter S (1985) Cited in Eisenburg N (ed.) Contemporary Topics in Developmental Psychology. New York: Wiley-Interscience, p. 286.

Harvey S (1980) The value of play in hospital. Paediatrician 9(8): 191–7.

Hayward R (1999) The present and future management of childhood craniopharyngioma. Child's Nervous System 15: 764–9.

Hazinski M (1992) In Ladig D, Van Schaik (eds) Nursing Care of the Critically Ill Child (2 edn). St Louis MO: Mosby, p. 10.

Hendrick J (1997) Legal Aspects of Child Health Care. London: Chapman & Hall, p. 238.

Hickey J (1992) Neurological and Neurosurgical Nursing. Philadelphia: JB Lippincott.

Hilderley L (1992) Radiation oncology: historical background and principles of teletherapy. In Hassey Dow K, Hilderley L (eds) Nursing Care in Radiation Oncology. Philadelphia: WB Saunders, pp. 3–16.

Holt F (1993) The role of the clinical nurse specialist in developing systems of health care delivery. Clinical Nurse Specialist 7(3): 140.

Hooker L (1999) Future trends. In Gibson F and Evans M (eds) Paediatric Oncology, Acute Nursing Care. London: Whurr, pp. 167–9.

Hooker L, Palmer S (1999) Administration of chemotherapy. In Gibson F, Evans M (eds) Paediatric Oncology, Acute Nursing Care. London: Whurr, pp. 22–58.

Hopkins M (1999) Tumours and radiotherapy treatment. In Gibson F, Evans M (eds) Paediatric Oncology, Acute Nursing Care. London: Whurr, pp. 423–32.

Hymovich DP, Roehnart JE (1989) Psychosocial consequences of childhood cancer. Seminars in Oncology Nursing 5(1): 56–62.

Jacoby A (1993) Quality of life and care in epilepsy. In Chadwick D, Baker G, Jacoby A (eds) Quality of Life and Quality of Care in Epilepsy: Update 1993. London: Royal Society of Medicine, pp. 66–78.

Johnson B (1995) One family's experience of head injury. Journal of Neuroscience Nursing 27(2): 113–18.

Kalifa C, Valteau D, Pizer B, Vassal G, Grill J, Hartmann O (1999) High dose chemotherapy in childhood brain tumours. Child's Nervous System 15: 498–505.

Kellie SJ (1999) Chemotherapy of central nervous system tumours in infants. Child's Nervous System Oct; 15(10): 592–612.

Kirke E, Howard V, Scott C (1995) Description of posterior fossa syndrome in children after posterior fossa brain surgery. Journal of Pediatric Oncology Nursing 12(4): 181–7.

Lefkowitz IB, Packer RJ, Ryan SG, Shah N, Alavi J, Rorke LB, Sutton LN, Schut L (1988) Late recurrence of primitive neuroectodermal tumor/medulloblastoma. Cancer 62: 826–30.

May L, Watson J (1999) Neurosurgery. In Gibson F, Evans M (eds) Paediatric Oncology: Acute Nursing Care. London: Whurr, pp. 318–61.

Mike V (1982) Incidence of second malignant neoplasms in children: results of an international study. The Lancet 2 (8311): 1326–31.

Moore I (1995) Central Nervous System toxicity in cancer therapy in children. Journal of Pediatric Oncology Nursing 12(4): 203–10.

Nadkarni TD, Rekate HL (1999) Pediatric intramedullary spinal cord tumours. Critical review of the literature. Child's Nervous System Jan; 15(1): 17–28.

Noll R, Pawletko T, Sulzbacher S (1993) Psychosocial support. In Albin AR (ed.) Supportive Care of Children with Cancer. Baltimore and London: Johns Hopkins.

Packer R (1999) Alternative treatments for childhood brain tumors. Child's Nervous System 15: 789–94.

Packer RJ, Sutton LN, Atkins TE, Radcliffe J, Brunin GR, D'Angio G, Seigal KR, Schut L (1989) A prospective study of cognitive function in children receiving whole brain radiotherapy and chemotherapy: two year results. Journal of Neurosurgery 70(5): 707–15.

Packer RJ, Sutton LN, Elterman R et al. (1994) Outcome of children with medulloblastoma treated with radiation, cisplatin, CCNU and vincristine chemotherapy. Journal of Neurosurgery 81: 690–8.

Phipps K (1996) A Retrospective Investigation into Long Term Educational Performance of Children treated for Medulloblastoma. University of Surrey. Unpublished BSc thesis.

Pollack IF, Boyett JM, Finlay JL (1999) Chemotherapy for high grade gliomas of childhood. Child's Nervous System 15: 529–44.

Reddy AT, Packer RJ (1999) Chemotherapy for low grade gliomas. Child's Nervous System Oct; 15(10): 506–13.

Ryan J, Shiminski-Maher T (1995a) Hydrocephalus and shunts in children with brain tumours. Journal of Pediatric Oncology Nursing 12(4): 223–39.

Ryan J, Shiminski-Maher T (1995b) Neuro-oncology nurses: Undaunted, hopeful, and enthusiastic. Journal of Pediatric Oncology Nursing 12(4): 179–81.

Shiminski-Maher T (1990) Brain tumours in childhood. Journal of Pediatric Heathcare 4: 122–30.

Shiminski-Maher T, Shields M (1995) Pediatric brain tumours: diagnosis and management. Journal of Pediatric Oncology Nursing 12(4): 188–98.

SIOP (1995) Guidelines for school/education. Medical Pediatric Oncology 25: 429–30.

Thompson J (1990) Sexuality: the adolescent and cancer. Nursing Standard 4(37): 26–8.

Tobias JS, Hayward RD (1989) Brain and spinal cord tumours in children. In Thomas DAF (ed.) Neuro Oncology. London: Edward Arnold.

Walker F, Roethke S, Martin G (1994) An overview of the rationale, process, and nursing implications of peripheral blood stem cell transplantation. Cancer Nursing 17(2): 141–8.

Wisoff JM, Epstein FJ (1994) Management of hydrocephalus in children with medulloblastoma: prognostic factors for shunting? Pediatric Neurosurgery 20(4): 250–47.

# Chapter 5
# Surgery for epilepsy

## Classification of epilepsy

Hippocrates (460–377 BC) was the first person to recognize epilepsy as an organic process of the brain. Many mystical explanations followed until the 1870s, when Hughlings Jackson suggested that seizures originated from a localized, discharging focus in the brain. The advent of the scalp electroencephalogram (EEG) by Berger in 1929 provided the first recordings of epileptic discharge from the human brain.

Epilepsy is a chronic condition characterized by seizures. Seizures can be defined as malfunctions of the brain's electrical system resulting from cortical neuronal discharge; however, the exact mechanism underlying this imbalance of inhibitory and excitory neurotransmitters, remains unclear. The manifestations of seizures are determined by the site of origin and may include loss of, or altered consciousness, involuntary movements, changes in perception, sensation and posture. Seizures can be induced by a number of acute medical or neurological conditions, including infections, drugs, hypoxia, hypoglycaemia and elevated temperature. Only when a number of seizures occur over a certain timescale can a patient be described as having epilepsy.

Epilepsy is the most common serious neurological disorder affecting people of all ages and occurs in 1 in 200 of the population (0.5%). Approximately 75–90% of all epilepsy has its onset before the age of 20 (Austin and McDermott, 1988). The most common ages of onset are between five and seven years of age, which implies that the immature brain is more prone to seizures, and also at the onset of puberty (Sands, 1982). The incidence of epilepsy rises again after the age of 65 due to vascular and degenerative disease.

The aetiology of epilepsy is variable but can be due to congenital or genetic reasons, prenatal (such as toxoplasmosis), traumatic (following head injury), infective (meningitis, encephalitis), neoplastic, vascular and idiopathic. Any person's brain has the capacity to produce a seizure if the conditions are right and in some individuals the seizure threshold may be lowered due to unusual stimulation, such as certain frequencies of flickering light or some drugs. Eighty per cent of children with epilepsy will achieve long-term freedom from seizures with anticonvulsant therapy, but the adverse effects of these drugs cannot be discounted. Seizure control by such drugs as phenobarbitone, for example, may contribute to poor developmental progress and behavioural and educational problems (Neville, 1996).

Epilepsy can be very broadly divided into two categories: idiopathic – where there are usually no other handicaps, the EEG is normal between seizures and response to drug treatment is good – and symptomatic epilepsy, which usually develops as a result of some structural abnormality of the brain, is associated with other abnormalities (intellectual delay, behavioural abnormalities) abnormal EEG and a variable response to drug treatment.

The pathophysiology of epilepsy is threefold:

- electrical discharges may arise from central areas within the brain that affect consciousness;
- electrical discharges may be restricted to one area of the cerebral cortex, producing manifestations characteristic of that particular anatomical focus;
- electrical discharges may begin in a localized area and spread and, if extensive, produce generalized clinical manifestations.

Seizures can be described as partial or generalized.

### Partial seizures

#### Simple partial seizures

There may be an aura or warning prior to the seizure and this may include visual or auditory disturbance or an unusual taste or smell. There is no loss of consciousness. Rhythmical twitching may occur and depends on the affected part of the brain.

#### Complex partial seizure

There may again be an aura. There is an impairment of consciousness. Aimless wandering and purposeless activities are typical, and lip smacking, screaming and swearing and plucking at clothes can occur. This type of seizure is usually temporal or frontal lobe in origin.

Partial seizures can progress to become secondary generalized seizures where both cerebral hemispheres are simultaneously affected by the seizure discharge.

## Generalized seizures

These seizures originate from both cerebral hemispheres. There is loss of consciousness.

### Tonic clonic seizures (grand mal)

Tonic implies muscle rigidity and clonic implies rhythmical jerking of muscles. The child may become cyanosed and be incontinent There will be a period of sleepiness/unconsciousness following this.

### Absence seizures (petit mal)

These generalized seizures are characterized by a momentary loss of consciousness, often mistaken for daydreaming. They last a few seconds, can occur up to 100 times a day, and although they cause no long-term harm to the brain, their frequency interrupts the child's learning and concentration. Atypical absences may also include a loss of muscle tone causing the child to fall forward on the floor.

### Myoclonic seizures

These seizures are characterized by short, sudden muscle contraction of limbs and trunk; this may lead to a fall.

### Status epilepticus

This describes an episode of prolonged seizure activity, or a number of fits in quick succession with little or no recovery time.

### Febrile convulsions

Febrile convulsions are most common between one and four years of age and are related to a pyrexia often associated with teething, ear infections and tonsillitis. The risk of recurrence after a single febrile convulsion in children varies widely, but is probably around 50% (Garret, 1986). The seizure may have tonic clonic, or clonic movements and usually lasts a couple of minutes. Febrile convulsions are not usually classified as epilepsy and most children who have them outgrow them naturally without any problems. However, a strong association between prolonged febrile convulsions and the later development of complex partial epilepsy, has led to early aggressive treatment of febrile convulsions and instigation of steps to prevent their occurrence.

## Prognosis

About 80% of people with chronic epilepsy become seizure free on anti-epileptic medication (Shorvon et al., 1987). Although the type of seizure is the major determinant of drug choice, for most children the decision will be influenced by the frequency and nature of adverse affects, the convenience of drug regimes and toxicity. Single drug therapy will achieve long-term remission in over 75% of cases (De Silva et al., 1989) and Carbamazapine or Epilim is effective in the majority of cases. However, the choice of drug is dependent on the type of epilepsy. Ideally, drugs should be introduced alone and adjusted until seizure control is achieved, or until the side effects from the drugs become intolerable. Only then should another drug be introduced, attention being paid to the possibility of drug interaction. There is considerable variation in drug handling between children of different ages and even between children of the same age; babies, for example, clear anticonvulsants from their bodies remarkably quickly. Plasma drug concentration levels need to be assessed, the aim of treatment being seizure control alongside steady appropriate plasma levels with minimal side effects.

Of the 20–25% of children in whom anticonvulsant therapy is ineffective, surgery may be an alternative for a small portion of this group.

# Developmental and psychosocial aspects of epilepsy

There is an increased number of psychosocial problems in children with epilepsy. The majority of children with controlled epilepsy are cognitively within the normal range, although the IQ is slightly lowered, at about 85–92 points. The main problem in children with mild epilepsy is attention deficit, leading to underachievement at school and overprotection, lowered expectation and low self esteem. Children with a long history of epilepsy frequently have memory difficulties affecting both working memory and new learning. Left-hemisphere pathology underlying seizures is associated with poor verbal skills and poor memory, whereas right-hemisphere pathology is associated with impaired visuospatial skills and visual memory. Children in whom seizures start in early childhood typically have poor language skills. Intractable epilepsy may be associated with cognitive decline. Prolonged periods of subclinical activity are also associated with cognitive decline and behavioural regression, even when there are few observable seizures. The fact that clinical and subclinical epilepsy may be directly causing developmental delay, arrest or regression, is pushing clinicians to earlier and more aggressive treatments as a preventative measure for such developmental impairments. Studies such as that by Kokkonen et al. (1997) and Jalava et al. (1997) highlight the long-term implications in terms of development and social issues, for the individual suffering epilepsy since childhood.

In addition to any neurological changes associated with seizures and the aetiology behind them, there is often a change in parenting behaviours for the child with epilepsy. Following a diagnosis of epilepsy, parents may react with fear, anger, guilt and sadness (Voeller and Rothenberg, 1973). Parents describe feelings of overwhelming disaster, along with concerns about behavioural problems and social handicaps.

The parent may be less confident in managing the child with epilepsy: the unpredictability of seizures causes unique stresses, parents and children experiencing a loss of control; disciplining the child may become a problem, with parents becoming over controlling or not exerting enough control over the child (Kessler, 1977). Family life is disrupted and parents expect more difficulties with the child. In addition, the view of society will influence parental attitude and coping. Parents and siblings have described feelings of embarrassment because of the stigma associated with epilepsy (Smith, 1978).

It is important for the professionals working with these families to assess parental attitude to their child in order to assist the parents in achieving a more positive attitude. The family's individual belief systems and evaluations need to be addressed as part of this assessment. Parents with a negative attitude towards their child's epilepsy, seem to develop poor coping strategies and are less able to seek support from others. The clinical nurse specialist and social worker can make contact with the family at the epilepsy clinic, providing support, education, resources and advice. They will liaise with the various professionals involved with the family within the hospital setting and the community to ensure good communication and continuity of care for the child and family.

## Treatment

### Dietary treatment

The ketogenic diet may be successful in controlling seizures, particularly in young children (Schwartz et al., 1983). Various different diets all appear to be as effective.

More recently, food allergies have been considered as a contributory cause of childhood epilepsy and a trial of 'oligoantigenic' or few foods diet, has been shown to improve seizures in 50% of children (Livingstone, 1991).The children in this study also suffered from migraine and the placebo effect of such diets must be considered.

## Steroids

There is little indication for the use of steroids in intractable childhood epilepsy, although some patients with Landau-Kleffner syndrome have shown some response (Livingstone, 1991).

## Immunoglobulins

Some long-term response to the use of immunoglobulins has been reported and further studies are warranted (Illum et al., 1990).

## Non pharmacological treatment

Precipitating or aggravating factors or causes should always be investigated; even with intractable epilepsy, there may be internal or external factors that stimulate seizure activity, and behavioural treatments have been introduced such as relaxation or biofeedback methods (Schotte and DuBois, 1989). Research is needed to evaluate these procedures more thoroughly.

## Surgical management of childhood epilepsy

The first successful surgery for uncontrollable seizures was described in 1886 (Horsley, 1886). Since that time, the introduction of anticonvulsant therapy has controlled seizure activity in the majority of patients; for those who continue to suffer an unacceptable number of seizures despite medication, or in whom the side effects of medication are unacceptable, surgery may be a possibility.

Until recent years, there has been a reticence about performing resective surgery for intractable seizures in young children; the reasons for this are twofold: first, because in the minds of both the physician and the parents, there is always a hope that seizures might resolve spontaneously; and second, the concern that damage may occur to the developing brain as a direct result of surgery (Peacock et al., 1993).

There is increasing evidence to suggest that seizures interfere with brain maturation, which results in delay or arrest in developmental milestones. Coupled with the suggestion that antiepileptic drugs may also interfere with cortical maturation (Diaz and Shields, 1981) the surgical option for the control of epilepsy becomes more acceptable. In addition, there is a greater understanding today of the normal history of the disease process. Improvements in patient selection and operative techniques have now made epilepsy surgery reasonably safe and successful, and consequently it is no longer viewed as such a high-risk alternative.

There are two types of surgery for epilepsy. The first is functional and is aimed at modifying seizure spread and is thus a palliative procedure; this includes multiple subpial transection and corpus callosotomy. The second is resective, the aim being curative by removing the epileptogenic process; this includes lesionectomy, temporal lobectomy, extratemporal resection and hemispherectomy.

A reduction in seizure activity means that the young child, in particular, has an increased opportunity to learn and develop to his or her optimum potential. Functional recovery is greatest in the young. After hemispherectomy for example, rapid changes are often noted in the young child soon after surgery, including the learning of new motor and vocal skills despite resection of the dominant hemisphere.

## Presurgical clinical evaluation

The goals of investigations of intractable seizures in childhood are to localize the epileptogenic focus and to assess the functional and structural normality of the tissue beyond resection.

Presurgical evaluation and investigations vary between units. A multidisciplinary team approach is taken to discuss each patient on completion of investigations, prior to making patient selection and surgical recommendations. The parents will be advised as to the anticipated outcome of surgery and any decisions taken will be in conjunction with them. Should their child be selected for surgery, many issues arise for them: the extent of the surgery and the inevitable or potential consequences associated with it; the responsibility of giving consent for surgery and putting their child at risk from potential complications, particularly if there is a question as to a successful outcome. The possibility of a real reduction or absence of seizures and the consequences of this often overwhelms them. A clinical nurse specialist (resources allowing), or another key professional, is an important link in ensuring good communication between the parents and the team, in listening to and understanding their fears, and in providing support, education and encouragement in reaching a decision regarding their child's future.

An extensive diagnostic work up precedes surgery, including electrophysiology, neuropsychology and imaging studies. All these studies should suggest an epileptogenic focus, for the child to be considered for surgery.

The investigations required include those listed below.

### Electroencephalography (EEG)

Electroencephalography is essential for identifying and analysing seizure activity and also for identifying a potentially resectable area. Abnormalities can be detected between seizures (interictally) and during seizures (ictally). Interictal spikes are helpful in localizing an epileptic area;

however, although seizures may begin in one area, interictal spikes may occur in multiple areas throughout the brain. It is therefore important to record EEG activity during a seizure to identify the area where seizure activity starts. In some centres, sphenoidal electrodes may be inserted immediately below the zygomatic arch to provide further information regarding seizure onset, although this is usually reserved for adult patients due to the invasiveness of the procedure. Whatever form of EEG is performed, seizure activity must be monitored at the same time; clinical behaviour and electrical changes will help localize the site of seizure activity, and video monitoring alongside continual EEG monitoring may be beneficial for some, but not all patients.

*Telemetry*

Specific telemetry areas have been set up to facilitate continuous EEG recording alongside video monitoring. Since medication may have been withdrawn prior to this investigation, appropriate nursing surveillance is essential to ensure patient safety. Therefore telemetry is best performed in designated telemetry units, where all staff are skilled in caring for the child and family undergoing telemetry. Professionals must be aware of any potential status epilepticus, bearing in mind that following withdrawal of medication, seizure activity will be increased and often unpredictable. Reassurance to both child and parent that the child will be kept safe during this time, is essential. In addition to keeping a written record, the nurse will have continual video coverage displayed at the nurses' station to ensure that the child is continually supervised. The usual care of the fitting child is applied, attention being given to the maintenance of the patient's airway and appropriate oxygenation in addition to preventing self harm.

*Invasive monitoring*

In many cases, scalp electrode EEG monitoring together with additional investigations (described below) are the most appropriate method of localizing seizure activity. However, recordings from the scalp surface do not always localize seizure activity of focal origin and consequently, in selective cases, EEG recording with intracranial electrodes may be performed. Subdural electrodes are used and although the information received from grid EEG recording when compared with scalp EEG recording can be much greater, patient selection is a major consideration. The most commonly used form of electrode type in paediatric monitoring is subdural grids or strips. The purpose of recording from grids is twofold: first, to document the presence and location of seizure discharges, and second, to locate functional cortex that the surgeon would wish to preserve, such as those areas responsible for language, sensory and motor function. By locating critical areas of cortex, a brain 'map' can be documented, and later used by the surgeon. Subdural grids provide extensive surface coverage without puncturing the brain (Rutkowski, 1990), but in some cases, depth electrodes are placed. These are directed deep into the brain cortex to record from either deep or superficial cortical structures.

In the past, surgeons have been reluctant to use grid implantation in the very young child as this was thought to hinder their development, although this is no longer perceived as true. Since earlier surgery is now thought to improve later psychological status and adaptive behaviour, and to increase the likelihood of achieving a functionally independent adult, surgery is being performed at an early age. This requires accurate assessment of seizure focus and brain anatomy and the possible need for intracranial electrodes to define this.

Grids can be placed using image guidance and therefore a preoperative MRI scan is required, although this can be done months before surgery. An initial craniotomy is required for insertion of the grids and a CT scan may be performed following surgery. The child is monitored with simultaneous EEG and videotape recording in the telemetry bay until adequate information is obtained, which is usually within seven to 14 days. Leads extend from the implanted grids to cables that attach to an amplifier. The EEG machine and computer record electrical activity 24 hours a day. Clearly for the child with behavioural difficulties, maintaining a secure head dressing over the wound site is of major concern and requires patience and skill from both nurse and parent. Although prophylactic antibiotics may be used postoperatively, infection remains a potential complication and one that can be significantly reduced if the child can be restrained from interfering with the dressing. Cerebrospinal fluid leakage may further increase the risk of infection, and in many centres, the dressings are reinforced rather than replaced, in an attempt to reduce the infection rate.

A hyperactive child with wires attached from the grids is also a challenge in terms of safety and security, requiring constant surveillance and supervision. Many of these children will not be compliant with bed rest for any period of time, and long cables attached to the grids will allow supervised activity around the cubicle. All monitoring equipment should be either wall mounted or well secured and nothing should obscure the view of the child from the video camera. Anticonvulsants may have been reduced or withdrawn to allow more seizures to occur, rendering the child agitated, irritable, and more prone to unpredictable seizures. Safety is a major issue during this time (Sanders et al., 1996) and the practice of family-centred care is essential in involving the parents and extended family in assisting with their child's care during this stressful time. Children with behavioural difficulties may respond better to their parents, who may have certain methods of calming their child or gaining their compliance. A good rapport between nurse and parent will result in improved communication and understanding. The nurse must gain the parents' confidence to ensure they take rest periods themselves during this difficult period; these parents are often highly skilled in the care of their child, understanding his or her unique needs and behaviour; consequently they often find it difficult to relinquish the child's care to others, even for a short period. They need to be reminded that, following this period of invasive monitoring, a further and more extensive craniotomy will be required to remove the grids and, hopefully, resect the area of seizure focus; they therefore need to pace themselves with regard to their own health, sleep and energy.

Invasive monitoring carries with it the aforementioned potential complication of infection: blood cultures, full blood count and CRP (C reactive protein) should be taken in line with hospital policy. In addition, bleeding, cerebral oedema, increased intracranial pressure, tissue trauma and anaesthetic reaction may occur following insertion of intracerebral electrodes. Any drowsiness or new neurological deficit should be reported and a CT scan considered. Vomiting may persist for the first day or two and antiemetics should be used. Appropriately trained medical and nursing teams are required throughout this period of monitoring.

Anticonvulsants may have to be discontinued in order that a number of habitual seizures are recorded (up to six is usually sufficient). A protocol should be in place outlining the treatment of seizures during the monitoring, to ensure accurate recordings of seizure activity while maintaining the child's safety. Functional mapping will then take place in an attempt to outline the seizure activity and focus. The child will normally proceed to surgery 10 days following grid insertion.

*Magnetic resonance imaging (MRI)*

Magnetic resonance imaging scanning, provides more sensitive pictures than CT for the detection of patients with refractory epilepsy. Abnormal signal activity, cerebral atrophy or lesions can be identified and the surgical procedure considered accordingly (Sperling et al., 1986). Due to the age, behaviour and cognitive nature of many of the children selected for surgery, sedation or general anaesthesia may be required for the scan.

*Functional imaging*

Single photon emission computerized tomography (SPECT) scans are physiological imaging studies that measure blood perfusion of the brain. A radioactive tracer (HMPAO) is administered intravenously, which diffuses across the brain–blood barrier. Single photon computerized emission tomography tracks the single photons resulting from radioactive decay using the gamma camera, which collects data from various angles to reconstruct regional blood flow. Continuous EEG monitoring, usually following drug withdrawal, allows the HMPAO to be administered and the presence of hyperperfusion (due to seizure activity) demonstrated. Ictal and interictal studies will be performed; recent studies suggest that the sensitivity of interictal SPECT is higher in adults than in children, but that these studies may still not be as reliable as ictal studies (Cross et al., 1995).

Children undergoing SPECT may have unpredictable and violent seizures following drug withdrawal; they may in fact be intentionally stimulated to have seizures, by means of undergoing strenuous activity on a springboard, or by sleep deprivation. Following extensive investigations, absence of seizure activity during this time can be frustrating for the family, who are keen to reach a decision regarding surgery. Nurses and parents must work in unison to ensure the child's safety during this time and at no time must the child be left unsupervised.

Positive emission tomography (PET) scans are physiological imaging studies that measure glucose uptake and metabolism, oxygen uptake, and cerebral blood flow patterns. A compound labelled with a positron-emitting radionuclide tag is injected into the patient. The compound selects concentrates in the areas of clinical interest and emits positrons. Photons are produced as the positrons decay, and their movement is detected by scanners; these data are collected in a computer, which reconstructs images of the labelled compounds. Positive emission tomography scanning provides the best of all the physiological imaging techniques, and although it is highly informative with regard to epilepsy, it is very expensive and available only in major research centres.

## Neuropsychology

Preoperative neuropsychological evaluation and testing is important in determining the location and extent of brain dysfunction. It provides a baseline for the child's level of functioning. In carrying out the neuropsychological assessment of a child with epilepsy, special attention is given to assessment of short-term memory due to the importance of the hippocampus and mesial temporal regions in memory formation; in addition, a range of standardized and experimental tests are used to provide information in the following areas of cognition:

- basic cognitive function such as IQ;
- memory: long term versus short term; verbal versus visual;
- receptive versus expressive language;
- visuospatial function;
- processing speed, attention, and executive functions;
- school attainment.

For the young child or those children with severe handicaps, developmental assessments need to be adapted accordingly.

Neuropsychological profiles help identify selective impairments in different aspects of cognitive function, and relate these to underlying focal pathology or lesions. These profiles are also examined to identify atypical forms of cerebral organization and/or reorganization.

Many children with epilepsy develop behaviour disorders, and hyperactivity is a common finding. Psychosocial, neurological and medication related factors all contribute to the behavioural, educational and cognitive outcome of the child with epilepsy.

A psychologist specializing in the treatment of children with epilepsy is also a source of guidance and advice for the family, who may be dealing with a child with multiple psychosocial difficulties. Some of these children display behaviour and language that is unacceptable in society; by understanding the reasons behind the behaviour, and recognizing triggers that may instigate it, the family may find mechanisms by which to diffuse the situation. The psychologist can also assist them in coping themselves, when dealing with the long-term issues related to their child.

# Surgery

### Focal resective surgery (temporal lobectomy)

In children with seizures arising from the temporal lobe, CT and MRI scans have shown a surgically resectable lesion in 80% of patients (Peacock et al., 1993); in the majority of cases, the hippocampus has been involved.

Focal resection is performed on patients with uncontrolled partial epilepsy, when the portion of the brain responsible for causing the seizures can be removed with minimal morbidity. This may include patients with sclerosis, gliomas, dysembryoplastic neuroectodermal tumours (DNETs) hamartomas or vascular abnormalities. Contraindications for this surgery include the presence of a neurodegenerative disorder, or seizures of multifocal origin. Seventy to 80% of patients become seizure free following temporal lobectomy (Spencer, 1986). Other benefits including psychological and rehabilitative status. Risks of surgery are small (Brewer and Sperling, 1988) but include visual field defects, dysphasia, third nerve palsy, hemiplegia, and infection.

Situated inferior to the temporal horn is the hippocampus, which is involved in emotional behaviour and memory; the role of the hippocampus in epilepsy surgery has been observed in numerous cases, epileptic lesions often giving rise to hippocampal sclerosis, with resulting memory deficits.

## Hemispherectomy

Hemispherectomy is used for seizure control in children with refractory epilepsy and extensive unilateral hemisphere disease. The selection criteria are as follows: intractable seizures, hemiplegia contralateral to the damaged hemisphere, and anatomical and physiological testing that confirms that the hemisphere ipsilateral to the damaged hemisphere is normal. Anatomical hemispherectomy describes removal of the entire hemisphere and may be associated with complications such as haemorrhage and hydrocephalus. Functional hemispherectomy is not associated with these complications; however, leaving large proportions of the hemisphere behind makes later interpretation of EEGs difficult; the disconnection process is also technically difficult, especially with a severely dysplastic hemisphere.

In the majority of cases, the affected hemisphere is already severely damaged, with resulting neurological deficits; these may include a hemiparesis and hemianopic visual field defects. Congenital abnormalities such as hemimegaencephaly or Sturge-Weber syndrome result in a damaged hemisphere and surgery may be indicated in the first few months of life. Contraindications for this surgery include marked bilateral lesions, seizures that originate in both hemispheres, or a localized epileptogenic structural lesion that could be approached in a more restricted manner.

Although hemispherectomy is clearly extensive surgery, the unique ability of the young brain to relearn tasks, reorganize important functions and reorganize (known as plasticity), renders hemispherectomy a safe surgical tool for those children with diffuse hemispheric involvement. Moreover, there is an 80–90% reduction in seizures following hemispherectomy and improved behavioural and cognitive status.

## Multiple subpial transections

The above operative procedure was designed to treat seizures that arise in unresectable areas of cortex such as the speech areas. Transections are made horizontally in the superficial cortex spaced at 5 cm intervals. The supposition is that this interrupts the horizontal spread of seizure activity, but at the same time preserves the vertical integrity of the functional cortex. While still controversial, this surgery may offer some benefits to children with Landau-Kleffner syndrome, which is characterized by regression of language with a possible origin within the speech centres of the brain, and an epileptiform EEG. The success of surgery remains difficult to evaluate.

### Corpus callosotomy (commissurotomy)

Incision of the corpus callosum is indicated for patients with primary generalized seizures. This includes atonic, tonic, clonic, some partial seizures with secondary generalization, and some multifocal seizure disorders. Disconnection of the corpus callosum is used to prevent the propagation of seizures rather than their initiation, and is therefore used for those children who are not candidates for standardized resective surgery. The most beneficial effect of corpus callosotomy section is seen in drop attacks ('kinetic seizures') and although other seizure types might persist following surgery, eliminating drop attacks can result in a much improved life quality with reduced secondary injury. Contraindications include the presence of a neurodegenerative disorder, or localized structural disorder. A reduction in seizures has been achieved in up to 75% of patients. Risks following corpus callosotomy include partial seizure activation or transformation, and long-term neuropsychological consequences such as manipulospatial dysfunction and hemispheric antagonism.

### Preoperative care

The time between assessment and admission for surgery can seem endless to the parents. Having been informed their child is a candidate for surgery raises expectations of a potential improvement in lifestyle for the child and the entire family. Parents' goals must be realistic and it is often useful to establish a 'contract' with them, ensuring their thorough understanding of the situation. The possibility of a reduction in seizure activity, or a seizure-free life for their child, is now a possibility, and the wait is difficult. The availability of a clinical nurse specialist in epilepsy, is of support and encouragement to the family, both before and following surgery. Having been offered surgery for their child, many parents are fearsome of the potential hazards of such major surgery, often without a guarantee of a successful outcome. An experienced specialist nurse can answer many questions that arise concerning surgery and alleviate some of the fears and concerns surrounding it.

Further discussion is often necessary at the time of consent for surgery, and when the reality of surgery is present. Parents may need reassurance that they are doing what is best for their child, in allowing him or her the chance for an improved lifestyle.

The preoperative care required is similar to that required for any craniotomy. A blood profile must be checked and adequate amounts of blood cross matched. Clotting studies must be performed to ensure that anticonvulsant medication has not altered the normal status.

Starvation prior to theatre will be in line with local protocols, but extra supervision may be required for the child with reduced understanding and/or lack of compliance, to ensure this is adhered to. Precautions should be taken such as removing all food and drink from the vicinity; explaining the dangers of eating during this fasting time to parents and gaining their assistance in supervising the child are also helpful. Anticonvulsant medication should be administered as prescribed to coincide with the last oral fluids taken.

Preparing the child psychologically for surgery should be undertaken in conjunction with the parents. They have a unique understanding of their child's comprehension and coping abilities, and can work alongside the play specialist or ward nurse in deciding on the most appropriate methods of explanation and preparation for their child. The adolescent patient with behavioural abnormalities, for example, can be difficult to manage, both in physical and psychological terms, and parents should be encouraged to use their knowledge of their child in defusing potentially difficult situations.

**Intraoperative care**

Epilepsy surgery has similar requirements to any major neurosurgical procedure. The operation may be lengthy and therefore attention given to avoiding pressure sores and hypothermia. Extensive surgery can result in large blood losses and rapid blood transfusion may be necessary, particularly in the very young child. Intraoperative EEG recording may be required and this will have been discussed and planned prior to operating.

**Postoperative care**

*Lobectomy and callosotomy*

The care requirements for these children are similar to those required following any craniotomy, raised intracranial pressure due to oedema or haemorrhage always being a possibility. Neurological assessment must be undertaken as appropriate and possible when caring for those children with severe behavioural abnormalities: pupil reaction may be impossible to assess, and experience and common sense are requisites of the nurse caring for these children; parents can be of assistance in confirming what is the normal behaviour and verbalization of their child, whose compliance may be improved (or not!) in the presence of the parents. In addition to the normal requirements of the child following craniotomy, there are specific requirements outlined below, which are specific when caring for the child following surgery for epilepsy. Many of these are associated with the child's cognitive and psychological state.

Maintenance of a patent airway is of paramount importance, particularly if seizures occur in the immediate postoperative period. These fits, though of great concern to the family, are generally a result of handling of the brain during surgery rather than an indication that surgery has failed; they do, however, require prompt action (Richardson, 1989) by means of anticonvulsants. The neurological status of the patient is closely monitored for signs of raised intracranial pressure and decreasing motor function.

Analgesia is given regularly. However, some of these children are unable to communicate their pain verbally, and the nurse's experience along with the parents' knowledge of the child are useful tools in assessing the child.

Blood replacement may be necessary postoperatively, particularly in the infant. Monitoring of vital signs and arterial monitoring will be undertaken according to local policy, though this will involve constant surveillance when caring for the hyperactive child, or the child with behavioural difficulties. Parents can be involved in supervision of the child in conjunction with the nurse, as they may often (but not always) gain better compliance from the child.

Intravenous fluids will be given until oral fluids are tolerated. This is often a difficult process as the child's behaviour may be such that he or she will not eat or drink when in a hospital environment; each child and family must be evaluated on an individual basis with regard to early discharge; the likelihood is that the child's behaviour will return to normal when in the home environment.

Anticonvulsant therapy must be continued and this can be done intravenously, rectally, or orally as appropriate. It may be difficult to gain the child's compliance when taking oral medication and, once again, the parents may be the most appropriate people to administer drugs, in the manner with which the child is familiar.

Redivac drains will be removed once drainage has decreased sufficiently; a full head dressing is advisable in the majority of these children, to reduce the risk of scratching and contaminating the wound. The presence of periorbital oedema will further irritate the child; patience and constant supervision are necessary, and need to be negotiated between parents and nurse.

Once recovered sufficiently, many of these children will rapidly become mobile, even within a day of surgery. It is tempting to allow very early discharge from hospital when this occurs, but it is not uncommon to experience a relapse in the form of lethargy or vomiting in the days following this period of hyperactivity.

Visual field defects may be a result of surgery and include a homonymous hemianopia, where the nasal vision in one eye, and the temporal half in the other, is affected. This is due to the visual pathways being cut during surgery. Such patients may be taught to turn their head to the affected side and thus improve their vision. Diplopia may also occur, but usually improves as cerebral oedema decreases in the days following surgery. Assessment of visual field defects is difficult in this group of children and may be more successfully achieved at a later date.

Dysphasia may be quite marked following surgery, but generally recovers completely without the need for speech therapy.

Memory defects are usually unremarkable, as preoperative measures are aimed at reducing the likelihood of such complications.

Neurological deficits may be expected, unexpected, temporary or permanent. If expected, the family will have been counselled beforehand, if unexpected, they require reassurance. Explanation will be required when a permanent and unexpected deficit occurs.

**Hemispherectomy**

In addition to the points described above, there are specific complications following hemispherectomy. Raised intracranial pressure is rarely a problem as there is excessive space caused by removal of such a large area of cerebrum. However, an aseptic meningitis is not uncommon, and the child can experience prolonged hyperpyrexia that can increase the likelihood of seizure activity, make the child feel very unwell, and increase parental anxiety. Antipyretics in the form of paracetamol and brufen, coupled with tepid sponging, are often enough to reduce the temperature sufficiently. Should hyperpyrexia persist over a few days, septic screening may be undertaken but is rarely productive in finding a cause, and the pyrexia eventually subsides spontaneously.

Vomiting can also be a persistent problem for days or occasionally weeks following hemispherectomy. Regular administration of antiemetics is undertaken, and the child supported with intravenous fluids as necessary. Plasma electrolytes need to be checked and maintained within normal limits during this time, and attention given to the route of administration of anticonvulsants: those that can be given rectally or intravenously should be done so, until it is evident the child is absorbing orally. Plasma anticonvulsant levels will confirm whether the correct drug requirement is being obtained and drug doses and administration routes can be altered accordingly. Drug assays, however, have not been developed for many anticonvulsants and are mainly available only for phenytoin, where compliance and drug toxicity may be an issue.

Lethargy and sleepiness are common following hemispherectomy, particularly in the adolescent patient. Frequent periods of rest are necessary between any treatments such as physiotherapy, and the family needs to be reassured that this is a common occurrence during this time. A CT scan may be performed when faced with prolonged sleepiness but this will rarely provide any evident cause.

In addition to the problems described, this group of children often has problems such as with gastric reflux, which flares up during all the alterations in medication and feeding. Hospitalization following hemispherectomy may therefore become extended and can last up to 14 days following surgery.

Hemiparesis will be apparent in varying degrees following hemispherectomy, but this is an expectation and will have been discussed with the parents (and child if appropriate) in the preoperative assessment stage. If hemiparesis was present as a presenting symptom preoperatively this may be unchanged following surgery, or occasionally slightly worse. Physiotherapy, later coupled with input from the occupational therapist, will enable the majority of children to regain acceptable mobility. Young children in particular are very versatile and adapt remarkably quickly to such a physical change.

Late onset hydrocephalus can occur in a proportion of children following hemispherectomy, requiring placement of a shunt.

### Subpial transections

In addition to the potential complications following craniotomy, children undergoing subpial transections have a higher risk of suffering an intracerebral haematoma, and cerebral oedema leading to a functional deficit. Neurological assessment will detect such an occurrence and a CT scan should be performed, followed by the relevant treatment. With success of surgery being difficult to assess, such potential complications need thorough discussion with the parents to allow an informed decision to be reached with regard to surgery.

## Follow up

The use of surgery in childhood epilepsy should take place within a multidisciplinary team. Many different clinicians will be involved in identifying pathology and predicting outcomes in the assessment stage. Skilled and specialized nursing, medical and psychosocial teams are required throughout the child's care. Good communication is essential throughout, to ensure optimum understanding of outcome for the child. Unrealistic expectations should be discussed prior to surgery being undertaken, and unrealized hopes should be voiced and discussed following surgery that has been less successful.

Centres specializing in surgery for childhood epilepsy will have their own protocols, but the majority will review the child six weeks following surgery in a joint surgery/neurology clinic, with neuropsychological testing. Over the course of the next three years, an annual assessment of the child will be performed, including MRI scanning with SPECT, visual fields assessment, neuropsychology and medication review.

A clinical nurse specialist/other key professional is essential in co-ordinating the complex planning and implementation of care required by these children. Such a nurse is also essential in the days and months following surgery, always working closely with the community team; if unsuccessful, there will be many issues that the parents will wish to address; if successful, the family will be facing a very different new lifestyle.

## A family's view

Luke was born following a full-term normal delivery and his development continued normally. At 15 months old, he suffered his first seizure, associated with pyrexia and vomiting. When he was three, he commenced speech therapy and his mother noticed that he seemed unable to play on his own. At four years old he developed afebrile seizures, lasting eight to nine minutes and occurring once or twice a week; he occasionally had a left Todd's paresis following seizures. The family lived abroad at this time, and a combination of anticonvulsants had some effect on his seizure activity.

Luke was nine when the family returned to the UK. He attended mainstream school and also had private tuition at home; however his short-term memory was poor, he had an attention span of about five minutes and he was eventually statemented. Luke continued to have frequent seizures, preceded by an aura of an unusual smell; he became anxious, aggressive, disinhibited and unable to share; severe bullying forced a change of school and life improved a little.

Luke presented as a potential surgical candidate, with temporal lobe epilepsy. His MRI scan showed right temporal lobe atrophy and right hippocampal sclerosis; telemetry demonstrated that seizures originated in the right frontotemporal region; he had no focal neurology except that his co-ordination was poorer on his left side.

A neuropsychological assessment showed Luke had a low verbal IQ, and that he had significant behavioural and learning difficulties; he was immature in terms of his social skills with a continuing tendency to temper tantrums and aggressive behaviour to other children; he was hyperactive and disruptive.

Luke's parents described the ordeal of being selected as a potential candidate for surgery, and awaiting confirmation: the assessment time was a 'nightmare', with Luke being disruptive and the investigations being invasive; the possibility that surgery might not be an option after all this, was too much to bear, and both parents felt highly stressed and anxious – 'I think we were a pain'.

Luke was selected as a candidate for surgery. His parents were told that surgery offered Luke a 60% to 70% chance of being totally seizure free, a 10% chance of having a reduction in seizure activity, a 1% risk that his seizures might become worse, a 1% risk of a hemiparesis and a 5% risk of a complication such as infection.

**Mum's view**

'Most of Luke's school chums accept the way he is, they're used to his fits, but they do get cross when he won't share sweets and things; he doesn't show any remorse when he's done something wrong, and that's hard'. Mum describes episodes of bullying that resulted in a change of school, which solved the problem.

Mum also says that his disinhibited behaviour can cause problems when they're out and that he's pretty hyperactive which is exhausting. She has become accustomed to dealing with other people's reactions to Luke and on the whole, she's pretty resilient. She describes Luke as also being anxious, immature but very affectionate; he prefers young people for company and doesn't maintain friendly contact with his peers. Although Luke could 'ride a bike, make tea, dress himself and be aware of danger', he still required constant supervision due to his hyperactivity and disruptive behaviour.

Once surgery was a possibility, there was never any doubt for both Luke's parents that this was the correct course of action. Schooling was becoming a struggle and as Luke became older so his behaviour was less acceptable to those around him. His mother had very little free time as Luke required constant supervision to prevent him getting into mischief, or hurting himself. Luke's father was still working abroad at the time and although Luke's grandparents were very supportive, most of the responsibility and care for Luke fell to his mother. Luke and his mother appeared to have a good relationship, often sharing jokes and stories, although Luke clearly relied heavily on his mother for reassurance, boundaries and guidance. She explained:

> He's a very anxious child and needs me to constantly reassure him; he has little confidence in his own ideas and is frightened by anything out of the ordinary; he's terrified of the idea of coming into hospital, I thought we wouldn't get him in here; that made me hesitate and question whether we were doing the right thing, but I knew we were.

The wait for surgery seemed endless to Luke's mother, 'like being offered a carrot and never getting it'. However, as the day for admission arrived, Luke's mother described how terrified she became, how everything was 'suddenly real'; she described the 'what if . . .' scenario, going through all the potential hazards of surgery. She tried to stay channelled on the end result, but felt more terrified as the day came closer.

When the family arrived on the ward for admission for surgery, Luke was so frightened that his behaviour was highly disruptive, so we allowed them to wander around and outside the hospital in an attempt to acclimatize him; this was fairly beneficial and Luke was a little more compliant on return.

## Luke's view

Previous to his admission for surgery, Luke would change his mind frequently about undergoing surgery, one day saying that he was happy to have an operation that would stop his fits and the following day changing his mind: 'My friends don't care if I have fits and nor do I; Mum and Dad want me to have this operation to stop the fits, so I suppose I'll have to; I don't want to though, I'm scared.'

Luke remained distressed throughout much of his time in hospital, often crying inconsolably. He had three seizures in the immediate period following surgery and his parents' stress levels hit the roof, despite reassurances from the team that this did not indicate failure of surgery, but merely irritation of the brain due to the surgery itself.

Luke became calmer once he was moved from the high dependency unit into the quietness of a cubicle, when he was receiving minimal observation and once we had given up persuading him to retain his head bandage! He occasionally ventured out of his cubicle and interacted with the younger patients on the ward.

He was discharged home five days following surgery, having had no further seizures.

Six months later, Luke and his mother reported that Luke was seizure free. Life for Luke and the whole family was much easier, with Luke gradually having more independence and an improved quality of life. His mother felt that he had more confidence in himself and that his schooling was 'taking off, though there's a lot of catching up to do'. Luke seemed cheerful, although very shy and reluctant to make eye contact; he became animated when describing how he'd gone to his first football match, and his mother was beaming as he talked. She described her anxieties in allowing Luke more independence, her pleasure in finding she had time to herself, her fears that the seizures might return. Overall, she was delighted at the improvement to their lives and grateful that Luke had been selected for surgery.

# References

Austin J, McDermott N (1988) Parental attitude of coping behaviours in families of children with epilepsy. Journal of Neuroscience Nursing 20 (3): 174–8.

Brewer K, Sperling M (1988) Neurosurgical treatment of intractable epilepsy. Journal of Neuroscience Nursing 20(6): 266–71.

Cross JH, Gordon I, Jackson GD (1995) Children with intractable focal epilepsy: ictal and interictal. HMPAO single photon emission computerised tomography. Developmental Medical Child Neurology. 37: 673–81.

De Silva M, McArdle B, McGowan M, Neville BGR, Johnson AL, Reynolds AH (1989) A prospective randomised trial in childhood epilepsy. In Charwich D (ed.) Fourth International Symposium on Sodium Valporate in Epilepsy. London: Royal Society of Medical Services, pp. 81–4.

Diaz J, Shields WD (1981) Effects of dipropylacetate on brain development. Annual of Neurology 10: 465–8.

Garret WR (1986) Ethosuxamide. In Taylor WJ, Caviness MHD (eds) A Textbook for the Clinical Application of Therapeutic Drug Monitoring. Irving TX: Abbot Laboratories, pp. 235–55.

Horsley V (1886) Brain surgery. British Medical Journal 2: 670–5.

Illum N, Taudorf K, Hielman C, et al. (1990) Intravenous immunoglobulin: a single-blind trial in children with Lennox Gastaut syndrome. Neuropediatrics 21: 87–90.

Jalava M, Sillanpaa M, Camfield P (1997) Social adjustment and competence 35 years after onset of childhood epilepsy: a prospective controlled study. Epilepsia 38(6): 708–15.

Kessler JW (1977) Parenting the handicapped child. Pediatric Annals 6(10): 654–61.

Kokkonen J, Kokkonen E, Saukkonen A, Pennanen P (1997) Psychosocial outcomes of young adults with epilepsy in childhood. JNNP 62: 265–8.

Livingstone J (1991) Management of intractable epilepsy. Archives of Disease in Childhood 66: 1454–6.

Neville B (1996) The paediatric issues in epilepsy surgery. The Great Ormond Street, Institute of Child Health London Experience. In Arzimanoglou A, Goutieres F (eds) Trends in Child Neurology. Paris: John Libbey Eurotext, pp. 21–7.

Peacock WJ, Comair Y, Hoffman J, Montes JL, Morrison E (1993) Special considerations for epilepsy surgery in childhood: In Engal J Jr (ed.) Surgical Treatment of the Epilepsies (2 edn). New York: Raven Press, pp. 541–7.

Richardson E (1989) Surgery for epilepsy. Nursing. 3(33): 3–24.

Rutkowski KL (1990) Grid implantation in seizure patients. AORN 52(5): 953–74.

Sanders P, Cysyk B, Alice-Bare M (1996) Safety in long term EEG/video monitoring. Journal of Neuroscience Nursing 28(5): 305–10.

Sands H (1982) Epilepsy: A Handbook for the Mental Health Professional. New York: Bruner/Mazel.

Schotte DE, DuBois MA (1989) Behavioural medicine approaches to enhancing seizure control in children with epilepsy. In: Hermann BP, Seidenberg M (eds) Childhood Epilepsies: Neuropsychological, Psychosocial and Intervention Aspects. Chichester: John Wiley, pp. 189–200.

Schwartz RH, Eaton J, Ainsley-Green A, Bower BD (1983) Ketogenic diets in the management of childhood epilepsy. In Rode FC (ed.) Research Progress in Epilepsy. London: Pitman, pp. 326–32.

Shorvon SD, Chadwich D, Galbraith A, Reynolds EH (1987) One drug for epilepsy. British Medical Journal 1: 474.

Smith LL (1978) Social work with epileptic patients. Health and Social Work 3(2): 158–74.

Spencer SS (1986) Surgical options for uncontrolled epilepsy. Neurology Clinician 4(3) 669–95.

Sperling MR, Wilson J, Engel J et al. (1986) Magnetic resonance imaging intractable partial epilepsy: correlative studies. Annual Neurology 20(1): 57–62.

Voeller K, Rothenberg M (1973) Psychological aspects of the management of seizures in children. Pediatrician 51(6): 1072–82.

Worthington JF (1990) Firestorm in the brain. Hopkins Medical News (Spring): 21–5.

# Chapter 6
# Paediatric head injury

## Introduction

Head injuries constitute a major health problem. An estimated 40,000 children a year are admitted to hospital in the UK with a head injury and this now ranks as the most common cause of death in childhood (Appleton, 1994) – 10% of all deaths in the 0–15 age group. Approximately two thirds of these fatalities occur at the scene of the accident and the remaining one third acquire secondary brain injury which then leads indirectly to their death (Dykes, 1989).

In addition, head injury remains a major source of handicap and disability. Mild head injury accounts for at least 65% of all head injuries, but lack of consensus about what constitutes a head injury, and unreliable statistics concerning severity and outcome, complicate research around this very complex process.

The diagnosis of head injury is made on the basis of a history of trauma to the head and corroborated by a physical examination. Head injuries in children vary according to the age of the child, a significant number occurring under one year of age. This includes the baby with birth trauma to the skull, and the baby with non-accidental injury – the pathology of the latter producing different pathological effects on the nervous system. The disproportionately larger and heavier heads of young children render them more likely to suffer a head injury. Falls on stairs and against furniture become common as children become mobile. Between the ages of four and eight years of age, injuries are more likely to be caused in road traffic accidents, on bicycles and in playgrounds; childhood head injuries are most prevalent during the summer months, when children are outside more frequently, or windows are left open during warm weather. The incidence of head injuries slowly increases until the mid teens, when there is a dramatic increase in incidence, and this is associated with motor vehicles and alcohol intoxication.

# Anatomical considerations

The outcome following head injury is thought to be more favourable in children than in adults: the greater compressibility of the child's brain coupled with the greater pliability of the young skull, enable better transmission of the energy generated by an impact. Other physiological differences in infancy that change the response of the brain to injury, include greater water content of the brain parenchyma, open fontanelle and patent sutures, lower brain/CSF ratio, lower ICP, different head/body ratio and compensatory mechanisms for blood loss (Thompson, 1999). The mechanism of trauma differs between adults and children. The brain injury following head trauma is more commonly a diffuse type in children, as opposed to the focal haematomas and contusions seen in the adult population, consequently the CT scan depicting a diffuse injury in a child will often appear superficially relatively normal. A history of a period of hypoxia or hypotension is often present in these cases and mortality rates can be very high.

Mild head injuries in children may often only include scalp lacerations and abrasions; at other times and in the absence of external signs, lethargy, vomiting and headache may be the only signs that head injury has occurred. Reduced concentration, sleep disturbance, memory dysfunction and double or blurred vision may also occur; these symptoms usually resolve spontaneously but can persist for up to a year following injury (Wade et al., 1998). Post concussion symptoms can cause significant psychosocial problems and often coincide with neuropsychological impairments, including memory dysfunction and speed of information processing (Dikmen et al., 1998). The Medical Disability Society recommends that all patients with head injury should be routinely followed up with an outpatient's appointment, and that includes the child with a minor head injury.

Head injuries may be open or closed injuries (depending whether the skin is lacerated or not) the latter being associated both with and without skull fractures. Thorough debridement of the scalp should always be undertaken. Fractures of the skull are found in approximately 30% of all paediatric head injuries although many are reported as normal by the doctor who first sees them. Skull fractures in children are not as predictive a factor with regard to the outcome following injury as in the adult. The skull fractures and splintering of the cranial sutures may, in fact, dissipate some of the impact energy and thus minimize brain injury. Severe head injury can occur in children in the absence of skull fractures, and clinical neurological status is a far more accurate indicator of intracranial pathology than plain X-rays.

'Growing fractures' are unique to children. A linear fracture with underlying dural damage can cause herniation through the dural tear. In the following weeks or months the fracture gradually grows, and there may be underlying areas of brain injury and leptomeningeal cysts, which push out and separate the edges of the sutures. Surveillance with CT scans and X-rays is required and surgical repair of the deficit may become necessary.

In all but the baby and young toddler, the cranium is a fused box with only one major opening at the base of the foramen magnum. The intracranial vault is smooth in some places and irregular in others. Major blood vessels running beneath these bones can be ruptured during trauma and an example of this is the middle meningeal artery. Fracture of the thin temporal bone overlying this artery may cause its rupture, and an epidural haematoma may result.

# Mechanisms of injury

Head injury can be divided into primary and secondary injury. Primary injury describes the initial mechanical injury to the brain and may be focal or diffuse. Diffuse injuries can vary enormously, according to the severity of primary impact and the shearing force exerted on the brain, with tearing of axons and small blood vessels. Patients who have sustained minor shearing injuries may have minimal long-term disabilities, whereas those with severe diffuse injuries are more likely to suffer significant morbidity and mortality.

Secondary injury describes the additional damage that follows the primary insult and which may lead to ischaemia and infarction. Secondary injury can occur immediately following the primary injury, or even days later. It can result from hypoxia, systemic hypotension and sustained raised intracranial pressure, as well as from the many metabolic changes that complicate multisystem trauma. These problems result in inadequate supplies of oxygen and nutrition to the brain that are essential for cell metabolism, and these factors contribute to poor patient outcome. Focal injuries include contusion, laceration and haemorrhage and once again, although the outcome is unpredictable, the severity of the injury gives some indication of the long-term outcome.

The pathophysiological changes associated with head injury are not fully understood. The main considerations are given below.

### Altered cerebral haemodynamics

Hypertension, hypotension and hypoxia increase the morbidity and mortality associated with severe head injury (Piugla et al., 1993).

The brain is vulnerable to deprivation of adequate cerebral blood flow (CBF) and cerebral oxygen delivery. Cerebral perfusion pressure (CPP) is the difference of the mean arterial pressure (MAP) and intracranial pressure (ICP), therefore a reduction in MAP would lead to a fall in CPP, thus exacerbating any existing brain injury. Therapy should be aimed at optimizing cerebral perfusion pressure:

$$CPP = MAP - ICP$$

Ideally the CPP should be maintained at > 60 mm Hg and this can be achieved by reducing the ICP, possibly combined with increasing the MAP. Various treatments are available to achieve these aims (discussed below); each of the treatments has limitations and the benefits of some remain to be proven.

### Hypercapnia

A rise in $CO_2$ (due to hypoventilation) increases hydrogen ion concentration. This exerts a local vasodilatory effect on the arterioles of the brain, which causes an increase in cerebral blood flow and consequently a rise in ICP. Hypocapnia conversely leads to vasoconstriction and may reduce ICP. Caution needs to be exercised if using this treatment as vasospasm and cerebral ischaemia can result.

### Cellular mechanism

Abnormally high levels of excitory neurotransmitters are found in the brain following head injury, in particular glutamate, which is known to be neurotoxic in high concentration. The increase in glutamate activates the inotropic glutamate receptor (NMDA) and metabotropic glutamate receptor (the G proteins), resulting in increased intracellular calcium. Disturbance in calcium homeostasis results in an increased breakdown of proteins and lipids, an increased breakdown of cell membranes, and the production of toxins, including free radicals. The outcome is oedema and cell death.

### Electrolyte disturbance

Hyponatraemia causes cerebral oedema with devastating morbidity and mortality. It can be caused by inappropriate antidiuretic hormone secretion or cerebral salt wasting, both of which can be triggered by an insult to the brain. Hyponatraemia and hypo-osmolality are a potent recipe for cerebral oedema.

Hyperglycaemia is also related to poor outcome following head injury. Hyperglycaemia in response to the stress of injury induces lactic acidosis and subsequent oxygen free radical production, which is detrimental to the injured brain tissue (Lam et al., 1991).

## Cerebral oedema

The degree of oedema is unpredictable and multifactoral. There are numerous causes – it may be a focal phenomenon in a contused brain, or a more global response to a diffuse injury. Continuous cycles of biochemical and vascular alterations further increase cerebral oedema, and irreversible neuronal changes and cell death may follow. Cerebral herniation may occur due to severely increased intracranial pressure.

## Cerebral ischaemia

Cerebral function can be profoundly altered by cerebral ischaemia. Ischaemic penumbra describes brain tissue characterized by compromised CBF between the upper limits of the threshold for electrical failure, and the lower limits of the threshold for membrane failure (Astrup, 1982). The clinical relevance of the penumbra is that the cells are still viable, and that tissue recovery is possible if an adequate blood supply is re-established. This concept provides a basis for potentially minimizing secondary brain injury.

## Pyrexia

For every degree Celsius increase in body temperature, there is a 5% increase in metabolic rate, which precedes an increase in cerebral blood flow (and ICP) in response to this increased activity (Arieff et al., 1992). Pyrexia also causes an insensible water loss which, if not corrected, predisposes to hypovolaemia and a reduction in MAP and CPP (Lam, 1999).

# Clinical evaluation

Head injury is often further complicated by injuries elsewhere in the body that may result in rapid hypovolaemia, requiring urgent intervention or surgery. However, for this to be a valuable intervention, cerebral protection is essential from the start; initial resuscitation and stabilization at the trauma scene and en route to hospital, have a profound effect on the outcome. Effective resuscitation involves ensuring that oxygenation and blood pressure is maintained. Adequate perfusion and oxygenation to the brain will assist in preventing secondary injury and promote optimal outcomes for the patient. Haemodynamic stability throughout the main organs of the body is also essential.

Emergency management includes establishing and maintaining a clear airway to allow adequate oxygen levels to reach the brain; intubation may be required, appropriate care being taken to prevent cervical injury/minimize existing cervical injury. An initial baseline neurological assessment is conducted to detect trends in neurological status; vital signs will also be taken and related to the neurological status and to other body functions. Early communication and liaison with the neurosurgical team is advantageous.

Children in particular can become rapidly physiologically unstable and ideally should not be transported without sufficient personnel and resuscitation equipment. Intubating a small, unstable child is not always an easy option, but should be carefully considered before an ambulance journey to a casualty or specialized centre. Early liaison between teams, including the neurosurgeons and intensitivists, is essential in ensuring the optimum outcome for the patient.

Level of consciousness is a sensitive indicator of neurological change. Assessing and monitoring the young, distressed child can be phenomenally difficult and ideally should be performed by someone skilled in paediatric care.

Michaud et al. (1992) found that the Glasgow Coma Score (GCS) 72 hours following head injury, especially with regard to the motor component, was a significantly better predictor of morbidity than was the initial assessment. Factors most predictive of survival/mortality included severity of total injuries, and pupillary responses in the emergency room.

# Treatment

The result of traumatic head injury is not a single pathological event but a series of pathophysiological events that vary in severity and over time. Adequate oxygen delivery and haemodynamic stability remain in the forefront of management. The aim of any treatment strategy is to avoid and actively treat the development of intracranial hypertension. Surgical mass lesions usually occur soon after the injury and, in general, the sooner they are removed, the better the outcome. The other pathophysiological processes that may be apparent on scan include oedema, contusions, focal ischaemia and hydrocephalus. Raised ICP will occur in 75% of all severely head-injured children and a delay in treating this may result in irreversible neurological deficit. These features may also evolve with time, and there should be a plan to rescan, should the child's condition deteriorate or fail to improve. Medical management of the head-injured child is aimed at reducing intracranial hypertension and ensuring adequate oxygenation; the following strategies are used for the child following severe head injury.

### Prophylactic hyperventilation

Hyperventilation is often used following head injury to reduce cerebral blood flow, thus reducing cerebral blood volume and intracranial pressure. Although hyperventilation is effective and easy to control, it can result in a decrease in cerebral blood flow with resulting cerebral ischaemia. Persistent hyperventilation may render the child sensitive to changes in arterial carbon dioxide levels, and tracheal suctioning must be performed skilfully to avoid arterial dilation and a further rise in intracranial pressure. Prophylactic hyperventilation in the presence of intracranial haemorrhage has been proven to be deleterious (Muizelaar et al., 1991). Most sources suggest hyperventilation is effective for about three to four days, although others state that 24 hours is the limit; whichever strategy is used, abrupt cessation of hyperventilation is recognized to be deleterious, with a rebound effect on intracranial pressure.

## Patient positioning

Elevating the head of the bed to 30 degrees facilitates venous return from the brain; venous return is further enhanced by maintaining the head of the patient in the neutral position, avoiding lateral neck flexion. Attention must be paid to the child's blood pressure and positioning should be assessed on an individual basis.

Avoiding placing the child in the prone position or with extreme hip flexion will help reduce the intra-abdominal or intrathoracic pressure, which could otherwise interfere with venous return and intracranial pressure.

## Intracranial pressure monitoring

In the sedated ventilated child, the normal clinical parameters are removed. In these circumstances, intracranial pressure monitoring aids in the early detection of changes in ICP.

## CSF fluid drainage

An external ventricular drain may be inserted and drainage of CSF used as a means of reducing ICP; it should be used in conjunction with intracranial pressure monitoring and unit protocols for drainage should be followed.

Although often used, the effectiveness of CSF drainage in these circumstances remains unproven.

## Diuretics

Diuretics are a temporary measure by which to reduce ICP.

The osmotic diuretic Mannitol is preferred for managing intracranial hypertension, provided that the brain–blood barrier is intact; it reduces intracerebral oedema and produces a diuresis. The assumption is that extracellular water is withdrawn from the brain, resulting in reduced brain volume. Plasma electrolytes and urine output must be carefully monitored, and the drug should be used with caution for children with cardiac or renal dysfunction. Loop diuretics such as frusemide may be used, but unlike mannitol, they do not reverse intracranial oedema directly. Although loop diuretics may have a place in reducing intracranial pressure, they also reduce blood pressure and can result in hypokalaemia and hypomagnesia.

### Fluid management

Current thinking is that restricting fluid input has a minimal effect on cerebral oedema and can cause hypotension (Hickey, 1997) and the important aim is to avoid dehydration and hypotension. Blood should be replaced where indicated and a combination of colloids/crystalloids can then be used to control the blood pressure.

### Sedation and neuromuscular blockade

Sedation is used as a means of limiting intracranial hypertension related to agitation, restlessness, interventions and asynchrony with mechanical ventilation. Benzodiazepines are commonly used as they do not affect the cerebral blood flow or the ICP. Midazolam is often used and has a sedative-hypnotic effect; the difficulty with using such drugs is that neurological assessment is not possible.

Neuromuscular blockade drugs are sometimes used to induce paralysis to counteract the increase in ICP associated with interventions such as ventilation, suctioning, dressings and turning. Drugs include pancuronium and vecuroneum; the complication of using these drugs is, again, difficulty in assessing the child's neurological status with regard to limb movement.

### Analgesia

Sedative medications do not provide pain relief and a continuous infusion of morphine should be used to provide analgesia. Pain can result in increased agitation and consequently a rise in ICP.

### Seizure management

Seizure activity or status epilepticus may not be immediately apparent due to the use of neuromuscular blocking agents; tachycardia, hypertension and a rise in ICP may suggest seizure activity, and an EEG performed to confirm diagnosis. Seizures can greatly increase the child's ICP and undetected seizures can thus cause secondary injury. Anticonvulsants should be administered and the child's condition continuously reassessed.

Approximately 20% of children with severe head injury will suffer seizures, which will often remain a long-term problem. Even if the child is seizure free in the immediate period following the trauma, seizures can occur up to two years later.

### Hyperthermia management

Aggressive management of hyperthermia is essential as the patient is at risk from inadequate oxygen supply at the cellular level and secondary injury. Hyperthermia can occur because of cerebral irritation due to haemorrhage, infection, damage to the hypothalamus and as result of drug use. Cooling measures are necessary, such as fans, cooling blankets or ice packs, and antipyretic drugs.

### Hypothermia

The National Acute Brain Injury Study on hyperthermia (Bullock et al., 1996) aims to establish if hypothermia at 32 °C to 34 °C improves the Glasgow Outcome Scale measurement at six months following head injury. Current thoughts on induced, controlled hypothermia vary, but moderate hypothermia (32 °C –34 °C) is thought to reduce cerebral metabolism without the problems associated with severe hypothermia, such as haemodynamic instability and cardiac arrhythmias.

### Jugular venous oxygen saturation monitoring

Cerebral perfusion pressure is known to be predictive in terms of clinical outcome. A reduction in CPP is associated with decreased jugular bulb venous saturation, which suggests a failure of cerebral blood flow to meet metabolic demand. Continuous monitoring of jugular venous oxygen saturation via an oximetric catheter inserted into the jugular bulb, may provide an early identification of cerebral hypoxia or ischaemia, although the validity of this technique is currently under debate.

## Care needs

The multidisciplinary team caring for the head-injured child need to be well versed in the protocols set out by their unit. They need to be familiar with assessing level of consciousness, neurological signs, brainstem reflexes and motor function, in addition to recognizing and appropriately treating the signs and symptoms outlined above. The care needs of these children are many and complex.

## Parents in the ITU setting

Parents need information and explanation. This needs to be simple and repeated – much of the initial information given will be forgotten. During the initial assessment and treatment of the child it may be impractical to allow parents to remain at the bedside; however, parents are often reassured to hear about the treatment their child is receiving because they interpret this to mean that the situation is not hopeless (Hazinsi, 1992). Families will look to the ITU staff for clues about their child's condition, interpreting staff behaviour and interventions. The nurse needs to provide information to the family that corrects misconceptions or validates concerns, and to find additional support for family members as appropriate (Plowfield, 1999).

## Nutrition

Although nutrition is not the immediate concern for the head-injured patient, early neurological recovery from head injury has been found to occur more rapidly when nutrition has been provided soon after the injury; however, in the majority of cases, nutrition is not adequately established until several days following injury (Gardner, 1986). The hypermetabolism that occurs following any body insult, is notably severe following head injury.

Hypermetabolism and hypercatabolism together increase the complications associated with head injury, and they include infections and skin breakdown. A degree of immunodeficiency will occur five to seven days following inadequate nutrition; decreased protein stores and a nonfunctioning gastrointestinal tract further complicate the issue.

Appropriate calorific intake needs to be insured. Nutritional adequacy is determined by calculating the total number of calories absorbed, and comparing it with the patient's expected energy expenditure, taking into account the extra requirements following severe trauma and head injury. Nutrition should therefore be established at the earliest possible time following injury, to provide optimum benefit for the patient. Enteral feeding should established where possible, parenteral nutrition being reserved for conditions where gut absorption is not possible. Care should be taken when passing feeding tubes, and orogastric rather than nasogastric tubes should be used if skull base fractures are present.

Once the child's condition allows, oral feeding should be reestablished. This may require input from the speech therapist, attention being given to any maxilla-facial trauma, the child's positioning during feeding and ability to swallow efficiently.

Bowel management is essential to avoid a rise in ICP associated with straining; stool softeners or laxatives should be used as necessary, and a bowel management programme instigated when appropriate.

## Physiotherapy

Chest physiotherapy is indicated where there are areas of consolidation or collapse; this may involve manual techniques to assist in clearing secretions with suction. Good pulmonary function is essential to oxygenation and therefore chest physiotherapy should be instigated early. Transient rises in ICP during physiotherapy should not deter efforts to maintain pulmonary function.

A physiotherapist specializing in neurology is the ideal person to treat the child, as soon as it is medically safe to do so after admission. She or he will assess the child's tone, range of movement and active movements (if not sedated). The physiotherapist will work with the nurses on a positioning programme if there are problems with the child's muscle tone. If the child presents with spasticity, limb splints may be used. These provide a long stretch, which assists in preventing contractures in muscles that could, if they persist, require orthopaedic intervention at a later date. The physiotherapist will also work alongside the parents, teaching them how to perform stretches and positioning. This has a dual purpose: The child will receive more therapy than the physiotherapist alone can offer, and the parents feel they are doing something useful for their child, and contributing to his or her rehabilitation.

When considered to be medically suitable, with a stable ICP, the physiotherapist will stand the child – even though he or she may still be intubated and ventilated. A suitable chair should also be provided to enable short periods of sitting. Resources may limit the frequency of physiotherapy visits and the ward nurses can work alongside the parents in continuing the programme set out by the physiotherapist.

Once the child has moved out of the ITU, the programme of physiotherapy will continue. Abnormal posturing may become more apparent in severe cases, and positioning and splinting may need to be reassessed. Even in the presence of a low coma scale, early mobilization is encouraged once the acute phase of injury has passed.

Maximal support may be required initially, with pillow supports while sitting, and two people assisting with standing. A standing frame may be used. Parents will often be distressed at the child's inability to do such a normal task as standing independently, and need encouragement to support their child. Postural hypotension can occur on standing if the child has had a prolonged period of bed rest, and it may be prudent to measure the blood pressure during the initial attempts at standing.

As the child's condition improves, the physiotherapist will be able to assess the longer term needs of the child and may refer him or her to the occupational therapist. Recovery is dependent on the site and severity of the brain injury; those children with a milder head injury will be transferred to their local hospital, whereas more severely injured children may be transferred to a rehabilitation unit if available. There they will receive input from specialist physiotherapists, doctors and nurses, alongside speech and language therapists, and psychologists.

### Psychosocial support

As the child's condition improves and ventilation is withdrawn, an early picture of the child's neurological status begins to appear. He or she may be extremely agitated as a result of pain, fear, increased intracranial pressure or cerebral irritation. The nurse is the best person to recognize changes in the child's neurological status and to separate these signs from those attributed to exhaustion and pain. Calm and efficient care is necessary, and parental involvement may be appropriate at this time. However, parents will suffer a multitude of emotions and this may hinder a positive input; each situation must be assessed individually.

Protecting the child from self harm forms a major part of the nurse's and parents' role while the child is in an agitated state. Cotsides on the bed and constant supervision are essential to ensure the child's safety. This state of agitation may be shortlived, but can be a more permanent state, depending on the degree of brain injury sustained. The child may hit out at people and become very violent and abusive; swearing is common and parents are often highly embarrassed about this. Boys may often play with their genitalia causing further embarrassment to those around them. In addition to the difficulties in dealing with the child's disabilities and difficult behaviour, the uncertainty of the long-term outcome adds further stress to the family. The unpredictability of the outcome and the waiting required to see this outcome, cause a feeling of helplessness and frustration for the family (Mishel, 1981). Encouraging early participation in their child's care may assist them in beginning to come to terms with the situation. Performing tasks also gives parents a sense of control; in a study by Plowfield (1999) families reported feeling more in control when nurses requested assistance with giving the patient medicine, decreasing their sense of agitation or reorientating them; families reported that any small task such as holding the child's hand was important in gaining a sense of control during these crises. In addition to the nurse, a social worker, psychologist, family therapist and chaplain can be of assistance. If the family feels supported and involved it will be able to provide a higher level of support for the child (Addison and Shah, 1999).

**Play**

In the fourth century BC, Aristotle believed that young children should not work as this was detrimental to their growth; he also believed that play was essential to healthy development. By the seventeenth century children were depicted in artwork as attempting to understand the adult world through play.

Anna Freud (1928) and Melanie Klein (1932) pioneered the use of play as a means of communication and emotional release for children; play therapy was later described by Lowenfield (1935); he suggested that play therapy offered a treatment approach for young children, who by nature of their age, were unable to communicate verbally.

The Save the Children Fund (1989) reported on the role of the play specialist. Hospital play specialists are educated to identify the child's current level of understanding and can initiate play that is interesting and diverse. The service provided by the play specialist is recognized as being distinct from nursing but the two team members will often work together in providing a catalyst for play.

Children with restricted mobility, impaired vision and communication difficulties can be provided with stimulation through play; this increases awareness and verbal activity, and helps prevent behaviour such as head banging and other self-injurious behaviour that can arise from understimulation.

Activities designed to promote sensory stimulation can be both enjoyable and educational. These include objects that have different textures, are visually stimulating and have different sounds and aromas. Once the child's condition is stable, visits to a multisensory room, if available, can be beneficial, providing a variety of sensory activities geared to the individual child, within a comforting and safe environment.

Basic play activities can involve simple measures such as holding the child closely, thus promoting the feeling of comfort and security. This may be resisted by the child in the early days following injury when handling and disturbing the child can increase cerebral irritation, and this can be distressing for the parent. Children enjoy close physical contact, and this enjoyment should return as the child's condition improves.

# Rehabilitation

Rehabilitation refers to the process of functional restoration and relearning. The goals of rehabilitation are to improve the quality of life, to optimize physical abilities, to promote health preservation and to decrease health service costs (Davies, 1985; Sherburne, 1986).

Rehabilitation of the head-injured child begins on admission. Involvement of the family unit in assisting and implementing care is vital,

including assessing needs of hygiene, stimulation, nutrition, physiotherapy and forward planning. Family involvement can help reduce the
feeling of helplessness and provide some degree of control over the situation, feeling helpless being a normal status for a parent. Early intervention
is usually based on physical rehabilitation and the emphasis subsequently
changes to encourage functional and intellectual recovery. The occupational therapist becomes involved at the rehabilitation stage, resources
permitting. The occupational therapist's aim is to attempt to rehabilitate
the child in terms of play, feeding, washing and other activities of daily
living. Specialist seating and wheelchairs may be required, and the
occupational therapist will need to liaise with the social worker and local
teams to access finance and resources. Returning to school is a goal for the
child and family, although cognitive problems may necessitate reassess-
ment of previous schooling; many occupational therapists are experts at
perceptual skills and this can be of particular assistance to those children
with a cognitive deficit. The educational psychologist and hospital school-
teacher, where available, will form part of the team assessing the child.
Input from a clinical psychologist can help the child and family deal with
behavioural problems: children are frequently aggressive following head
injury and this may be partly due to their difficulty in understanding and
being understood; this behaviour may last for weeks or longer and
coupled with verbally abusive language can make the situation very hard
for the family and carers.

Nurses working with children require an in-depth knowledge of
normal growth and development, and their skills must be related to
physical, cognitive and psychological aspects (Greenwood, 1994). It is
essential that nurses teach the family to be involved in their child's care,
and they must also meet the family's needs. Self-care and independence
are promoted as they would be in normal childhood development, but
many families may need encouragement to develop this. Nurses are often
pivotal in co-ordinating the child's complex care and can often form
beneficial relationships with the child and family. Empowering families of
the ill child and providing integrated care pathways will lead to improved
outcomes for the child and family.

The expected outcome for this group of children will be that they can
maintain their own respiration and nutrition and that they become as
responsive and orientated as their condition allows. The expectation is
that their recovery progresses and that goals set in conjunction and participation with their family are realistic and achievable. Fulfilling the goals of
rehabilitation will reduce the stress levels for the family and help them
regain a meaningful life. Goals must be set in conjunction with the parents
and community team, to ensure continuity of the child's programme of

rehabilitation. Early liaison between hospital and community will decipher what assistance the community can offer in the form of nursing, physiotherapy, occupational therapy, social worker and so forth.

The child's condition may necessitate transfer to a rehabilitation unit prior to discharge home. Such units provide skilled, trained staff, cost-effective rehabilitation and a therapeutic environment within a continuum of rehabilitation, from early intervention until integration back into the community.

## Outcome

The outcome for very young children with severe head injury is worse than that for toddlers and older children and this is probably related to the cause and pathophysiology of the injury. Non-accidental head injury is common in the under twos and delay in requesting medical attention and treatment results in hypoxia, ischaemia and a poor outcome.

Predictors of poor outcome for accidental trauma in children include multiple trauma, shock and early hypoxia. The GCS, applied soon after injury, can also be a predictor of outcome (Levin et al., 1992). Mortality rates in children remain high, being 10% or even zero when children have presented with coma scales of five. Morbidity following paediatric trauma varies according to the outcome measures used. Scott-Jupp et al. (1992) found that 42% of head-injured children in their study had persistent neurological impairment, and 35% required special schooling, 13 months following severe head-injury. An increased incidence of psychiatric disturbance is present, even after minor injuries, with the family describing the child as 'just not the same'. Severe head injury almost always results in some measurable alteration in cerebral function, be it cognitive, neurological, social or psychiatric. Long-term memory and short-term memory are often affected and this can be extremely disruptive for the child and family.

Sleep disturbances and difficulties at school increase the problems faced by the family (Tepas et al., 1990). Normal patterns of family interactions and family structure are changed and family members find that physiological changes are easier to accept than personality or behavioural changes in their child (Hickey, 1997). Rivara et al. (1992) estimated that in 50% of the families he studied there were high levels of stress and disrupted family relationships, particularly among those families whose child had suffered a severe head injury. However, as in many studies regarding family coping mechanisms when a child becomes ill, Rivara et al. found that preinjury coping was a good predictor of postinjury stress. The multidisciplinary team must identify those families most at risk; an early understanding of family dynamics and functioning will help identify such families and enable optimum support to be provided (May and Carter, 1994).

## The future

The aim of care should be prevention. Diamond and Maccioch (1998) describe the need for a strategy for educating the primary care teams with regard to prevention methods. Government policy is being directed towards accident prevention, enabling people to make an informed choice about their health (Mackintosh, 1991); however, this policy is often not implemented, for example with regard to cyclists, where VAT increases the already high price of cycle helmets and the provision of cycle lanes remains minimal (Clayton, 1997). Cycle accidents are the most common causes of head injury in children and studies have shown that this can be reduced by up to 85% by the wearing of cycle helmets (Di Scala et al., 1991). Road safety and safe cycling practice also need to be addressed. Government policy and campaigns with the help of motoring associations, parental education and co-operation and school involvement, must be the way forward in preventing road accidents.

The lack of clinical trials makes it difficult to impose rigorous management guidelines for the head-injured child. Therapy for the treatment of paediatric head injury should be based on studies of recovery, rather than on those based on mortality. A consistent tool for measuring morbidity would allow accurate measures of recovery to be compared and thus shared, ensuring optimum treatment for these children.

## Non accidental injury (NAI)

Any child under the age of two presenting with a head injury should be evaluated with regard to having suffered an NAI and taking into account that the injury suffered might be due to deliberate injury by a parent or carer. Due to the presence of an open fontanelle and patent sutures, the classic signs of raised intracranial pressure may not be present. All medical and nursing staff should be familiar with the Trust's child protection policy and procedures so that appropriate measures are undertaken immediately.

Brain injury caused by NAI can be due to violent shaking, blows to the head, strangulation, and throwing the child with force against a surface. The child may have been repeatedly injured over a period of time, and cigarette burns to the child's skin may be apparent; X-rays may reveal sternal fractures of differing ages. In the absence of any external injury, the child may be brought to casualty with a history of vomiting, irritability and, sometimes, seizures; alternatively, such children may be transported by ambulance, their parents/carers reporting that they found them cyanosed and had revived them by shaking them. Presentation and patterns of injuries that should give rise to concern include a serious head injury following reportedly minor trauma, subdural or subarachnoid haemorrhage, retinal haemorrhage, injuries of different ages and injuries that are inconsistent with the child's development. Subdural haemorrhage is the commonest form of NAI found on neurosurgical units and is an unusual occurrence following accidental injuries in children; retinal haemorrhage is found in 90% of shaking injuries and, in the presence of a subdural haemorrhage, is strongly suggestive of NAI.

The child's immediate needs may include resuscitation, seizure control and blood transfusion. Burr holes may be performed through which the subdural bleeds can be intermittently tapped as required, a temporary subdural shunt being performed at a later date if needed. Brain injury can be severe and death can occur; less severe injury can result in various degrees of neurological damage, including developmental delay, epilepsy and blindness.

Where NAI is suspected, the consultant and senior nurse responsible for the ward must be informed of the child's admission; the social worker must also be contacted and this includes an out-of-hours contact, according to Trust protocol. Other professionals involved with the child should include a consultant paediatric neurologist, who will co-ordinate medical investigations into possible physical abuse alongside other medical colleagues and the social worker, a consultant neuroradiologist who may alert physicians to the presence of abnormalities suggestive of NAI, and a consultant ophthalmologist who will examine the child for the presence of retinal haemorrhages or other ocular injury. Communication between professionals and the parents is essential, as is good documentation. Where NAI is suspected, it may be necessary to obtain the child's obstetric notes relating to the child's delivery and postnatal care; this should include information regarding neonatal administration of vitamin K. Previous measurements of the child's head circumference are important in determining the time of onset of chronic subdural collections. A family history should be taken which includes details regarding any bleeding disorders, osteogenesis perfecta (including a family history of deafness), cot death and any injury to siblings (including step siblings).

Professionals may be reluctant to bring about or be involved in a process that will be distressing to the parents, and that could involve separation of the child from the family. Investigations should be fair, with the parents having an opportunity to present their own account of events. The social worker and if necessary the police will ultimately decide on the outcome for the child and in only a few cases will the child be removed from the family and placed in foster care. Many families will be allowed to take the child home if and when its condition allows under the supervision of the social services. Should investigations and procedures not be thorough, repeated injury could occur to the child with a fatal outcome.

Caring for these children can be emotive, particularly if the child is severely injured or in pain. A professional approach is necessary from all staff and a support network should be put in place for those caring for the child and family.

## An adult's reflections following head injury

Individuals have various memories of the accident or early rehabilitation; most memories involve the time immediately prior to the accident and then very little for a considerable time following that. However, in *Coma Reflections* (Paul and Littlejohns, 1994) a 23-year-old patient, recovering from head injury, recalls her memories of the early stages. Her memories provide a valuable insight into understanding the head-injured patient, and we should use her reflections to improve our own care.

She recalls a doctor 'being very concerned with this guy named ICP' and was distressed as she thought her own initials were MP and that they were discussing the wrong person. She remembers how everyone got excited 'when ICP was 19 or 20' and then someone would come into the room, and her relatives would start watching the 'TV' (monitors) next to her. Everyone seemed concerned about the 'ICP guy', and it was much later before the patient realized they were discussing her intracranial pressure! She describes how she just wanted to sleep and was immensely irritated with everyone trying to wake her up; she would have done anything to stop the doctors 'bouncing me violently on the bed and trying to wake me up'. People told her to do a 'thumbs up' and she couldn't do it; in rehab, she constantly made the 'thumbs up' sign, which she felt had become a reflex to questioning. Noises were also an irritation, and that included the 'accordion type machine . . . with a red plastic top' (her ventilator). She felt she would never be able to sleep 'with all this beeping and sooshing sound going on . . . the sound would get magnified in my head. The smell, it smelt like stale artificial air.' She describes being always scared if her mother or sister were not in the room with her. Nothing bad could happen if they were there. During rehabilitation, she feared sleep as she though she might go into a coma again and never wake up.

She describes her memory of the year and a half before the crash as patchy, and her current memory is poor, which frustrates her. She summarizes:

I know I'll never be the same as before, and I accept that now . . . I used to make things happen, now I have to ask for the simplest things to be done for me . . . I'm writing this so someone can learn from my experiences. I want to think my life has a positive meaning and something good will come from all this.

# A family's view

### Mum's view

Julie was a happy 12 year old, a sociable, popular child, doing well at school. Julie's mother was a paediatric nurse, currently working in a district general hospital. Julie was hit by a motorbike outside her house; her sister saw the accident and fetched their mother. Julie initially spoke to her mother, who consequently assumed the accident was not too serious. Julie said she was taken to the casualty department at the hospital where her mother worked.

Her mother describes how shocked she was, but how she failed to realize how seriously Julie had been injured until her level of consciousness rapidly deteriorated in the casualty department. Julie was intubated and ventilated; a CT scan was performed, which mother recalls as being frightening as the realization of the seriousness of the situation began to sink in. Julie was transferred to a paediatric intensive care unit in another hospital. Mum travelled in the ambulance with Julie for the transfer and says she went into 'nurse mode'; her daughter didn't look like her daughter and she felt she was transferring someone else's child.

Julie's mother describes everything on the ITU as a dream; she remembers very little detail, apart from the ventilator, lots of tubes and a child that she didn't recognize as her own. It was not until Julie was being weaned from the ventilator and making spontaneous movements and facial expressions, that her mother 'recognized her'. During their time on ITU, mum 'selected' nurses who she liked and felt confident with. She remembers episodes of anger when she shouted at nurses who she felt were not giving care at the correct time, or in a way that did not meet with her approval. She was also irritated that she was asked to leave the beside during doctors' ward rounds; she could understand why it was not appropriate to hear about the child in the next bed, but she saw no reason why she should not hear discussions about her own child.

Julie had an ICP probe in site; the ICP would rise when the ward environment was noisy, mum would massage her daughter, and the pressure would drop a little. A nurse told mum that some children could reach an ICP pressure of 80 cm and survive, but when Julie's pressure reached 50, the neurosurgeons requested another scan. Julie was taken for a craniotomy for evacuation of a frontal haematoma. Twenty-four hours later her ICP again climbed and she was taken back to theatre and her bone flap removed. She improved rapidly following this and was extubated two days later.

Julie spoke very soon following extubation and so it was a huge shock when she then became excessively agitated, irritable and aphasic. Mum says no one told her initially that it was common for a child's condition to fluctuate in this manner following a severe head injury. This was the first time that her mother had thought about the potential long-term consequences, rather than just the survival of her daughter. She decided that if her daughter was going to be brain damaged, she wanted her to be both physically and mentally damaged, so that she had no awareness of her own condition. She felt very frightened. She didn't want any visitors as she could not bear them to see Julie like that. She remembers her husband's distress and how calm and gentle he was with Julie. She felt that her nursing background gave her a perspective and understanding about Julie's condition that was different from her husband's, and so she wasn't sure if they both had the same thoughts in the early days.

Julie's mother initially didn't want anyone performing care for Julie as this increased her daughter's distress; she felt angry with the physiotherapists who started to mobilize Julie and stand her up, very soon following her transfer to the neurosurgical ward. Although it was explained to her why this was necessary, Julie's mother continued to find it distressing when her daughter had physiotherapy treatment or nursing care. She was encouraged to help with Julie's care, and to take support and encouragement from the team. She began to work alongside people, and to take some 'time out' for herself. She would not, however, leave the cubicle unless her husband or sister were there, so that if Julie was awake there would always be a face she recognized beside her.

Initially, on transfer out of ITU, Julie had found noise of any sort distressing but this phase passed rapidly. The only method of calming her during this early stage of rehabilitation was the playing of a 'tranquillity' tape.

Julie recovered rapidly: her speech returned over a period of days, she appeared to understand what her parents were saying and her physical status gradually improved. She was transferred to her local hospital (to the ward where her mother worked!) and was discharged a few weeks later. She returned to mainstream school the following term, where she remained in the same year, but with 'a few minor difficulties'.

Nine months later, Julie was readmitted to the neurosurgical ward for a titanium plate to be fitted. Although much of the detail above was gained from letter correspondence with Julie's mother, during this more recent admission she talked quite openly about her memories and feelings. Working on a paediatric ward, she encounters children who have not recovered from trauma to the extent that Julie has. She feels anxious when meeting these families initially, but is sure that her own experience enhances her care; she expresses empathy for the emotions they are going through, although is she constantly reminded of how fortunate Julie is.

She found the experience of writing down her feelings and talking about them at a later date to be cathartic. Finally, she told me:

> You know when parents are really traumatized and incredibly tired, they don't think about eating; you encourage them to take a break, go off the ward, get something to eat. They don't want to, so you tell them 'there's tea and toast available in the kitchen – help yourself.' When that was me, nothing in the world could have given me the energy or motivation to firstly get to the kitchen, secondly talk to anyone I encountered, or thirdly get my act together enough to make toast! So when I'm working and I recognize a parent who's in that state, I make them tea and toast and leave it in the cubicle. They always eat it. It's part of my care to that family. One less thing for them to handle in those early days of despair and exhaustion.

### Julie's story

Julie remembers what she was doing up until the time of the accident, but nothing at all for some time afterwards. Surprisingly, she enjoyed her time on the neurosurgical ward, liking the attention from the nurses and the constant presence of her parents! She has no unpleasant memories at all, and no recollections of invasive procedures or activities. She returned to the ward several months following discharge and seemed unperturbed by the environment and pleased to see familiar faces.

Her mother made her a scrapbook 'in case she had any recollections in the future'. Julie took the book into school and her parents feel this helped with her reintegration back into normal life. It also helped her friends and teachers to understand what had happened to her, and they felt able to talk about their own feelings of fear and uncertainty during Julie's hospitalization.

When Julie was readmitted for her titanium plate to be fitted, she was delighted to be back on the ward, apparently undisturbed by the experience. She proudly showed us her scrapbook, which included photographs of her time in intensive care and her rehabilitation, along with cards and messages sent by her school friends.

Julie appeared to be a well-adjusted and cheerful child.

# References

Addison C, Shah S (1999) Neurosurgery. In Guerreo D (ed.) Neuro-oncology for Nurses. London: Whurr.

Appleton R (1994) Head injury rehabilitation for children. Nursing Times 90 (22): 29–30.

Arieff AI, Ayus JC, Fraser CI (1992) Hyponatraemia or death and permanent brain damage in healthy children. British Medical Journal 304: 1218–22.

Astrup J (1982) Energy-requiring cell functions in the ischaemic brain. Journal of Neurosurgery 56: 482.

Bruce D, Trumble E, Steers J (1999) Pathophysiology and treatment of severe head injuries in children. In Choux M, Di Ricco C, Hockley A, Walker M (eds) Paediatric Neurosurgery. New York: Churchill Livingstone.

Bullock R, Chestnut R, Clifton G et al. (1996) Guidelines for Management of Severe Head Injury. New York: Brain Trauma Foundation.

Clayton M (1997) Encouraging children to use cycle helmets. Paediatric Nursing 10 (3): 14–16.

Davies A (1995) Focus on rehabilitation in the acute setting: the role of the clinical nurse specialist. Journal of Neurosurgical Nursing 17(3): 244–6.

Diamond PT, Maccioch SW (1998) Head injury – a survey in prevention health care counselling. Brain Injury 12(10): 817–20.

Dikmen S, Temkin N, Armsden A (1998) Neuropsychological recovery; the relationship to pyschosocial functioning and post concussional complaints. In Levin H, Eisenberg HM, Benton AL (eds) Mild Head Injury. New York: Oxford University Press.

Di Scala et al. (1991) Children with traumatic head injury: morbidity and post-acute treatment. Archive of Physical Medical Rehabilitation 72: 662–6.

Dykes J (1989) Evaluation of pediatric trauma care in Ontario. Journal of Trauma 29: 724–9.

Freud A (1928) Introduction to the Techniques of Child Analysis. New York: Nervous and Mental Disease Publishing. Cited in Gragam P (1986) Child Psychiatry: A Developmental Approach (2 edn). Oxford: Oxford Medical Publications.

Gardner D (1986) Acute management of the head injured adult. Nursing Clinics of North America 21: 555–61.

Godbole K, Berbiglia V, Goddard A (1991) A head injured patient: calorific needs, clinical progress and nursing care priorities. Journal of Neuroscience Nursing 23(5): 290–2.

Greenwood I (1994) The aims of paediatric rehabilitation. Paediatric Nursing 6(9): 21–3.

Hazinski M (1992) Nursing Care of the Critically Ill Child. St Louis MO: Mosby.

Hickey JV. (1997) The Clinical Practice of Neurological and Neuromedical Nursing. Philadelphia PA: Lippicott and Co.

Klein M (1932) The Psychoanalysis of Children. London: Hogarth Press.

Lam AM, Winn HR, Cullen BF, Sunling N (1991) Hyperglycaemia and neurological outcome in patients with head injury. Journal of Neurosurgery 75: 545–51.

Lam WH (1999) Mechanisms and management of paediatric head injury. Care of the Crtitically Ill. June 15(3): 95–8.

Levin HS, Aldrich EF, Saydjari C (1992) Severe head injury in children: experience of the traumatic coma data bank. Neurosurgery 31: 435–43.

Lowenfield M (1935) Play in Childhood. London: Gollancz. Cited in Black D and Coottrell D (eds) (1993) Child and Adolescent Psychiatry. London: Royal College of Psychiatrists.

Mackintosh N (1991) Self-empowerment in health promotion: a realistic target. British Journal of Nursing 4(21): 1273–8.

Martin K (1994) When the nurse says 'he's just not right'. Patient cues used by expert nurses to identify mild head injury. Journal of Neuroscience Nursing 26(4): 210–18.

May L, Carter B (1994) Nursing support and care: meeting the needs of the child with altered cerebral function. In Carter B, Dearmun A (eds) Child Health Care Nursing. Oxford: Blackwell Science.

Michaud LJ, Rivara F, Grady MS, Reay DT (1992) Predictors of survival and severity of disablement after severe brain injury. Neurosurgery 31(2): 254–6.

Mishel MH (1981) The measurement of uncertainty. Nursing Research 30: 258–63.

Muizelaar JP, Marmarou A, Ward JD et al. (1991) Adverse effects of prolonged hyperventilation in patients with severe head injury: a randomised clinical trial. Journal of Neurosurgery 75: 731–9.

Piugla FA, Wald SL, Shackford SR, Vane DW (1993) The effect of hypotension and hypoxia on children with severe head injuries. Journal of Pediatric Surgery 28(30): 31–6.

Plowfield L (1999) Waiting following neurological crisis. Journal of Neuroscience Nursing 31(4): 231–8.

Rivara JB, Fay JC, Jaffe KM, Polissar NL, Shurtleef HA, Martin KM (1992) Predictors of family functioning one year following traumatic head injury in children. Archives of Physical Medical Rehabilitation 73(10): 899–910.

Save the Children Fund (1989) Hospital; a deprived environment for children? The case for hospital playschemes. London: Save the Children Fund.

Scott-Jupp R, Marlow N, Seddon N, Rosenbloom L (1992) Rehabilitation and outcome following severe head injury. Archives of Disability in Childhood 67(2): 222–6.

Sherburne E (1986) A rehabilitation protocol for the neuroscience intensive care unit. Journal of Neuroscience Nursing 18(3): 140–5.

Tepas J, Di Scala C, Ramenofsky M, Barlow B (1990) Mortality and head injury: the pediatric perspective. Journal of Pediatric Surgery 25(1): 25–92.

Thompson D (1999) Head Injuries in Children; Head and Tails. The A and E letter. London: The Royal Society of Medicine Press Ltd, pp. 6–8.

Wade DT, King NS, Wendon FJ, Crawford S, Caldwell FB (1998) Routine follow up after head injury: a second randomised controlled trial. Journal of Neurosurgical Psychiatry 65: 177–83.

# Chapter 7
# Craniosynostosis

## Introduction

Craniosynostosis is not a new disease. There are references throughout history to the unusual head shapes, now recognized to be craniosynostosis. It is since the early 1980s, however, that enormous progress has been made in both the diagnosis and treatment of craniosynostosis. This has been made possible by the pioneering work of the French plastic surgeon Paul Tessier and also by the advent of improved scanning equipment, intraoperative techniques and medical and nursing expertise.

Normal growth of the skull vault occurs along the suture lines that separate one plate of bone from another. Craniosynostosis describes the premature fusion of one or more of these cranial sutures, and the resulting abnormal skull shape. The cosmetic result will vary between a minor abnormality, to one involving the whole craniofacial skeleton. The cosmetic abnormality will become more pronounced as the child grows, and regular clinical evaluation is necessary throughout childhood.

The recent discovery of the genes responsible for craniosynostosis is increasing understanding of the problems of progressive suture fusion. A greater understanding will also address the reasons behind developmental delay in some cases, and the presence of intracranial hypertension.

A multidisciplinary approach to the care of children with craniosynostosis is necessary to ensure optimum cosmetic and functional results.

## Types of craniosynostosis

The weight of the infant brain doubles in the first year of life and the skull must enlarge to accommodate this growth. When a cranial suture fuses prematurely, the law of Virchow (Virchow, 1851) states that the growth of the skull in the direction perpendicular to the suture will be reduced. However, in addition to the direct effect of the suture involved, there are further factors that contribute to the overall picture; they include the compensatory growth of the normal sutures, the presence of raised intracranial pressure, and the abnormal bone activity at cellular level in syndromic children.

A small proportion of craniosynostosis cases occur secondary to some underlying disease such as a haematological, biochemical or drug-related cause; the majority however are a primary anomaly.

### Single suture/non-syndromic craniosynostosis

Sagittal craniosynostosis or scaphocephaly accounts for 40% of cases of craniosynostosis. Fusion of the sagittal suture results in a long, narrow skull and frontal bossing. Early diagnosis and surgery results in optimum cosmetic results.

Coronal synostosis accounts for 25% of all cases. Unicoronal synostosis, or plagiocephaly, causes flattening of the frontal bone and a high rise of the sphenoidal ridge on the affected side; the supraorbital ridge is also affected. Unicoronal synostosis is often associated with a squint and head tilt. Bilateral coronal synostosis results in a short, high head, known as brachycephaly or turricephaly. It is most commonly seen in cases of syndromic synostosis.

Fusion of the metopic suture is known as trigonocephaly and accounts for 10% to 20% of all cases. The abnormality can be quite severe and is occasionally associated with certain genetic syndromes.

Lambdoid suture synostosis causes a flattening of one side of the occiput and accounts for 3% of cases. Posterior plagiocephaly however (which looks similar but has no premature suture fusion) is extremely common, and may be due to positional moulding – a response to lying in the supine position in utero. Both conditions are associated with torticollis and head tilt but, in posterior plagiocephaly, this appears to resolve spontaneously. Posterior plagiocephaly can result from the positioning of the young baby. Since the introduction of positioning of newborn infants and avoiding the prone position in relation to sudden infant death syndrome (SIDS), there has been a marked increase in the incidence of posterior plagiocephaly. The cosmetic abnormality may often spontaneously resolve, or improve with different positioning of the infant. Surgery for correction is rarely necessary.

### Syndromic craniosynostosis

#### Crouzon's syndrome

This is an autosomal dominant syndrome and the incidence is 1 in 25,000 births (Lajeunie et al., 1999). Crouzon's syndrome comprises

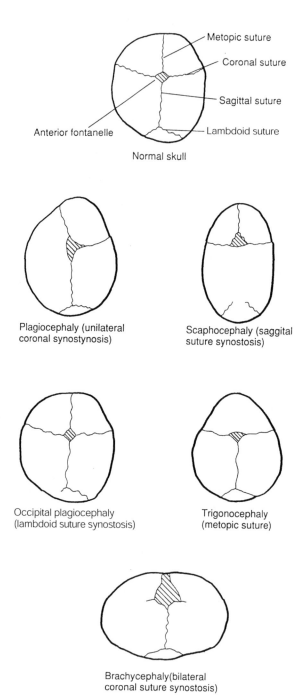

Figure 7.1. Craniosynostosis.

craniosynostosis, maxillary hypoplasia and proptosis. Although the features may be mild at birth they will progress and coarsen as the child grows. The coronal sutures are the commonest sutures involved and strabismus and a beak-shaped nose are also associated with the syndrome. There is a high incidence of raised intracranial pressure (Thompson et al., 1995).

### Apert's syndrome

This is also an autosomal dominant syndrome, most cases occurring as a fresh mutation. The frequency of this syndrome is 1 in 55,000 births (Lajeunie et al., 1999). Advanced paternal age may be a risk factor (Blank, 1960). Apert's syndrome involves synostosis of the coronal sutures and may involve some or all of the remaining sutures. There is hypertelorism, maxillary hypoplasia and sometimes a high arched palate with dental malocclusion and resulting respiratory complications. Syndactyly of hands and feet is a characteristic feature.

Abnormalities of brain development are also present – in particular hydrocephalus.

### Saethre-Chotzen syndrome

Brachcephaly is usually present although the abnormality may be asymmetrical, resulting in plagiocephaly and facial scoliosis. Mild syndactyly may be present, affecting the second and third digits in hands and feet.

### Pfeiffer's syndrome

This syndrome shares many similar features to those found in Apert's syndrome. There may be mild syndactyly, but, more commonly, the digits are unusually broad. The severity of the syndrome is variable, but includes those children with clover-leaf skull deformity.

### Clover-leaf skull (Kleeblattschadel)

This is a descriptive term and not a single syndrome entity itself. Synostosis of coronal, metopic and lambdoid sutures contributes to the severity of this abnormality and the trefoil skull shape. There is severe proptosis, and midfacial deficiency leading to upper airways obstruction. Raised intracranial pressure and compromised intracranial venous drainage further complicate the child's management.

## Clinical evaluation

Presuming the baby does not require immediate resuscitation, an assessment period will be necessary to decide the optimum care for the child and consideration should be given to the most appropriate setting for this to take place. Treatment may occur locally but more often the child is referred to a specialist centre, which is more familiar with the individual child's requirements. During discussions between parents and doctors, a nurse will be a valuable asset – particularly one who can provide time, support and initial information to the family, in addition to that provided by the doctor. The care requirements of the baby are variable, complex and involve the whole multidisciplinary team.

The main areas to be considered are respiratory, feeding, vision and intracranial hypertension, and consideration of these may need to take precedence over any cosmetic requirements.

Respiratory difficulties are most commonly seen in the syndromic forms of craniosynostosis. They are usually due to the narrow nasal and postnasal air passages, choanal atresia or maxillary hypoplasia. The ENT team and maxillofacial team will be involved at an early stage to assess and treat the individual child. The use of respiratory sleep studies has demonstrated obstructive sleep apnoea often accompanied by periods of raised intracranial pressure. This may be demonstrated by the use of intracranial pressure monitoring in conjunction with sleep studies (see ICP monitoring in Chapter 2 on hydrocephalus). The initial treatment may be the insertion of nasal stents and very occasionally the formation of a tracheostomy. Recently, the use of nocturnal continuous positive airway pressure (CPAP) has been beneficial for this group of children (Gonzalez et al., 1996) and can be used at home for those children who tolerate the mask. In later life, this group of children may require surgery to correct the midfacial hypoplasia.

Feeding may be difficult due to many of the same structural abnormalities that cause respiratory difficulties. Abnormalities of palatal shape and movement may necessitate the use of nasogastric or occasionally gastrostomy feeding. The dietician will be involved to ensure correct nutrition and weight gain, and the speech and language team will need to assess and treat oropharyngeal function and later, speech development. These difficulties may resolve as the child grows.

Vision can be impaired initially due to proptosis caused by shallow orbital sockets, which results in corneal abrasions and, in the more serious cases, prolapse of the globe. Early surgery may be necessary to bring the forehead forward and thus protect the eyes. In addition, impaired vision may be caused by optic atrophy in the presence of raised intracranial pressure; surgery to relieve the pressure may be required at an early age. The ophthalmic team will regularly assess and treat these children, both at diagnosis and throughout the child's continuing care.

Raised intracranial pressure is present in at least one third of children with craniosynostosis and is one of the main indications for surgery

(Thompson et al., 1994). Respiratory obstruction, hydrocephalus and impaired venous drainage appear to be causative factors and intracranial pressure monitoring is a useful diagnostic tool.

The diagnosis of hydrocephalus is complicated by the abnormal shape of the ventricles in many children with craniosynostosis. Signs and symptoms of raised intracranial pressure must be used in conjunction with ventricular size, to ascertain the presence of hydrocephalus; a ventricular peritoneal shunt will be the treatment required.

A geneticist will confirm any syndrome present and offer advice to the parents as to the possibility of any future children inheriting the same syndrome; he or she will also offer advice to affected children when appropriate, with regard to the risks for their own future progeny.

In addition to specific investigations required by the teams discussed above, plain skull X-rays will be necessary. A CT scan will also be performed with bone window settings if available, thus providing soft tissue and bone images, along with ventricular size. Intracranial pressure monitoring may be required. Photographs are taken to provide a baseline for future assessments.

The multidisciplinary team needs to assess each child as an individual and to make a treatment plan accordingly. The neurosurgeon and plastic surgeon will establish what degree of reconstructive surgery will be needed and at what age this surgery should be performed. Such information can be overwhelming and confusing to parents and the presence of a co-ordinator or clinical nurse specialist is highly beneficial. In addition to providing information regarding clinical requirements, this individual can be a central point of information for the parents, while also providing them with support and advice.

## Psychological evaluation

The initial shock to the parents when they first see their baby can be enormous, and the professional management of such a traumatic event can have a major influence on the ability of the family to cope with the child's condition (Burton, 1975). Staff may also be quite shocked by the baby's appearance and often feel uncertain what to say or do, particularly when faced with severe abnormalities such as the clover-leaf deformity. This behaviour is unhelpful for the parents who may be encouraged by seeing others handle and interact with their baby in a normal fashion. Babies with facial disfigurement are at a higher risk than those of normal appearance of developing an insecure attachment; the main determinant of secure attachment seems to be the mother's sensitivity and responsiveness to her infant (Crittenden and Ainsworth, 1989). From the time of birth, the mother of a baby born with a facial abnormality may be less 'available' to her baby. Langois and Sawin (1981) found that at two days old, less attractive babies are held less close and given less physical contact than infants seen to be attractive. In another study, Barden et al. (1989) studied mothers of facially disfigured children and mothers of infants of normal facial appearance at four months of age. He found that the former group behaved in a consistently less nurturant manner than those in the latter group, but were themselves unaware of any such difficulties. Surprisingly, they rated their satisfaction with parenting more positively on self-report measures.

This pattern of behaviour clearly does not apply to all parents whose children are born with a facial disfigurement; however, for those who do face attachment difficulties the future wellbeing of both infant and parent will be affected. Early recognition and intervention by a professional, be it the midwife, ward nurse, clinical nurse specialist, social worker, psychologist, doctor, or anyone with the understanding and experience to help can prove highly beneficial. Encouraging a more positive style of interaction between mother and infant, while giving the mother the time and understanding that she needs, can help promote a more rewarding and emotionally nurturing environment. An emotionally secure child will find it easier to form friendships and relationships and to have a higher self esteem.

Parents may have concerns about what the future holds for the baby and for the whole family. They may feel anger at the situation and non-acceptance of the situation or even of the baby itself; they may feel guilty that this has been caused by an event during pregnancy; they may feel saddened at the potential difficulties that lie ahead for their child. These issues need to be recognized and addressed at an early stage.

## Preoperative care

Once the family has been given a treatment plan and has understood the degree of surgical correction the that team hopes to achieve, surgery can be planned. Presuming there are no immediate problems requiring intervention, surgery will be planned selectively.

Preparation of the older child for admission for surgery can be undertaken with assistance from the ward play specialist and nurses in conjunction with the parents. Books, drawings and explanation can all help alleviate some of the child's fears and fantasies.

Most children with craniosynostosis are healthy children and require only the usual paediatric checks prior to surgery. A haemoglobin check and blood profile will be undertaken. Adequate blood should be cross

matched as the scalp is highly vascular, the operative exposure is extensive, and surgery can be protracted. The anaesthetist will assess the baby in
the usual way, giving special attention to the potential hazards that could
arise due to airway abnormalities. Some babies with Apert's syndrome, for
example, have large tongues and may be safer nursed in such a position
that their tongues fall naturally forward from the mouth following anaesthesia, thus avoiding partial airway obstruction. Discussion between
anaesthetist and parent will highlight the degree of any existing difficulty.

Surgical correction for craniosynostsosis is a major operation and
possible complications will be discussed in more detail with the parents
when consent is obtained for surgery. The ward nurse should be present
during these discussions to ensure that the parents have understood the
discussion and have had time to ask any questions. It is then possible for
the nurse to later reiterate what the surgeon has actually said, as parents
may have difficulty in grasping all the facts at an emotional time. Signing
the consent form often raises concerns and anxieties for the parents, who
may at this time, once again consider the ethics of putting their child
through what is for many, cosmetic, but major surgery.

## Postoperative care

The child will be nursed in a high-dependency setting/ITU/general ward
according to hospital protocol and the condition of the child.

On first seeing their child the parents will be distressed by its appearance however well they have been prepared. It is helpful if, during this
time, there is someone to comfort the parents and take them slightly away
from the bedside if possible. This allows the ward nurses to concentrate
on the immediate clinical needs of the child while it is still sleepy from the
anaesthetic, and this includes securing lines and drains. If the child is
already wide awake he may require his mother by the bedside; each family
and clinical situation should be assessed individually.

In addition to the usual needs, such as maintenance of airway and
positioning, the immediate requirements for these children include
analgesia and blood replacement. Analgesia will include a combination of
codeine phosphate, diclofenic and paracetamol and, if given regularly,
these children show remarkably little distress due to pain. Blood loss will
have been replaced intraoperatively but can continue through the redivac
drains in large volumes postoperatively and also, less obviously, subcuta-
neously. A replacement protocol for blood loss should be in place to
enable immediate blood or blood product replacement by the nurse; a
haematocrit and haemoglobin should be checked and this can be done at
ward level using an I-stat or similar blood gas machine if available; clotting

studies should also be undertaken if blood loss continues and FFP (fresh frozen plasma) given if required.

The patient should be monitored as for all major surgery, arterial monitoring minimizing disturbance to the patient by providing arterial pressure monitoring and blood sampling. All children with arterial lines should be very closely supervised at all times for safety reasons.

As the majority of these children are well, healthy children, their postoperative recovery is rapid. Vomiting may occur initially and the child should be supported with intravenous fluids until oral feeding is re-established. Prophylactic antibiotics may be prescribed for 48 hours postoperatively, in accordance with local policy. Periorbital oedema can cause distress and will become more apparent following removal of the redivac drains 24–48 hours postoperatively. Nursing the child in an upright position and the use of cold eye packs will help reduce the swelling. The child will need much reassurance during this time as the eyes may be totally closed; parents can hug and stroke their child to help soothe him; anyone approaching the child must talk to him prior to touching him; he will need to fed if unable to see. Boredom can soon set in and story and musical tapes, reading and tactile play, can be provided by the play therapist and nurse in conjunction with the parents in an attempt to relieve this. Parents must be given 'time out' at this tiring time.

Most children are able to be up and about within a few days, and home within a week of surgery, sometimes sooner. Normal feeding will have been re-established by this time and the nursing staff will advise parents with regards to the first bath and hairwash following surgery. Children's hair can be washed a few days following surgery. Sutures will be removed seven to 10 days post operatively and this can be done locally if this is more convenient for the family. The community team will be updated and informed of discharge instructions and future plans for the child.

## Discharge

The multidisciplinary team within the hospital and community will promote maximum physical recovery and improvement, and offer psychological support and understanding to the child and the family. Good communication is essential and should be co-ordinated through a central professional who is able to act in a link/liaison capacity – the clinical nurse specialist being the optimum person. Teachers and local social workers may need help to understand the sequelae of disfigurement and be educated accordingly.

The child should be well enough to return to normal activities on going home. However, major bumps and knocks should be avoided as much as possible – a challenge when dealing with a toddler! Minor bumps should not cause a problem but it is advisable to keep the child away from playgroup for a couple of weeks. Care should also be taken with the school-aged child and the child should be allowed to stay in the classroom at breaktimes and pursue quieter activities until reviewed in the outpatients clinic approximately eight weeks following discharge from hospital. Sports should also be avoided during this time.

# The future

### Future surgery

Children with craniofacial dysostosis syndromes such as Crouzon's syndrome and Apert's syndrome will have more complex requirements because the facial bones will also have been affected and this may require further major surgery in the future. The timing of this surgery is on an individual basis, although the ideal time is at about 16 years of age when bone growth is complete. Earlier surgery may be dictated by such functional problems as feeding or dislocation of the eyes.

When surgery is carried out before bone growth is complete it is often necessary to carry out a further operation at the end of the adolescent period in order to position the teeth properly. Operations to move the facial bones forward are called Le Fort osteotomies. The Le Fort I involves moving the tooth-bearing part of the upper jaw forward; the Le Fort II involves the above in addition to surgery to the nose; the Le Fort III involves advancement of the whole of the upper jaw, nose, cheekbones and eye sockets forward; the Le Fort III may sometimes be extended into the skull to move the forehead forward and this is known as a monobloc advancement. This latter procedure can dramatically improve the child's appearance. Occasionally a facial bipartition will be performed and the face split vertically along the nasal bridge, thus bringing the eyes closer together, expanding the upper jaw and rotating the two halves of the face into a more normal position. The latter procedure is reserved for the extreme cases of syndromic craniosynostosis.

### Hand anomalies associated with craniofacial conditions

The most severe hand abnormality is that associated with Apert's syndrome, although there are milder anomalies associated with Pfeiffer's syndrome and Saethre-Chotzen syndrome. Children with craniofacial conditions may undergo many operations for their craniofacial anomalies; the main priority of hand surgery is therefore to provide the child with as fully functional a hand as possible in one operation. The more complex the anomaly, the more surgical procedures are necessary.

The child's overall condition permitting, commencement of surgery will be at about four months of age when both hands may be operated upon during one surgical episode. If surgery is performed on the hands separately, operations can be carried out at three-monthly intervals. Surgical approaches vary but the main aim is to have good functioning hands, with as many separated digits as possible.

Postoperatively, the hands are kept constantly elevated for the first 24 hours and then during the day for a further three to five days. This helps reduce haemorrhage, oedema and pain. Two weeks following surgery, the dressings are changed and this is performed under general anaesthesia due to the fragility of the skin grafts; further dressings are performed on the ward at one to two weekly intervals until healing is complete in about six weeks. The incision lines should then be massaged with a moisturizing cream for about 18 months to promote a good final result and a flat, soft scar. A pressure garment or 'glove' will be provided by the physiotherapist, which will enhance the final cosmetic result; this glove will be worn for 23 out of 24 hours a day for about a year. Support splints may also be necessary following osteotomies. Children are very adept at using their hands soon after surgery despite their inability to bend their fingers.

In the long term, fine movements such as doing up buttons will always be difficult, although children are very versatile. Despite advances in surgical techniques, many children will be left with abnormal hands; encouragement and praise are helpful and necessary, and practical measures such as Velcro fastenings give the child added confidence and independence.

### Future care requirements for the child with craniosynostosis

For the child with a simple form of craniosynostosis, the degree of facial disfigurement is minimal and a single operation will often be all that is required. For the child with facial dysostosis, who may have other abnormalities in addition to facial disfigurement, there may be frequent hospital visits, operations, and a higher level of psychological disturbance to both the child and family.

As with many children who have repeated hospital admissions, the child with complex craniosynostosis may form an attachment to hospital, and a sense of dependence results. Hospital can be viewed as the 'family'. Although this can reflect the nurturing and 'safe' environment offered by the hospital staff, it is not always a healthy perception to harbour for life. Integration back into society should be encouraged and promoted in a positive fashion by all the multidisciplinary team.

Short-term psychological needs involve assessment of family functioning, of developmental and intellectual functioning, of behavioural and emotional status and of self esteem and schooling. Overprotection by parents means such children may fail to have normal childhood experiences that would prepare them for adult life. Real fears and anxieties need to be addressed but parents should encourage their child to reach independence and autonomy as far as possible. Teasing, rejection and social isolation at school can occur, resulting in withdrawal by the child, reduced learning capacity and overprotection by the parents. The school needs to be involved in dealing with any bullying and teasing and the child can be encouraged to develop coping skills. The psychologist can help the child learn non-aggressive assertion skills that will be helpful throughout life (Bradley, 1997). Siblings can also be the recipients of teasing and bullying and should be helped accordingly. They may feel jealous of the attention their sibling receives from the parent and this needs to be recognized and addressed.

Long-term needs involve intervention based on the effectiveness of treatment offered. This includes the child's/parents' satisfaction with the complete care they have received. Training for other professionals in the field and raising public awareness and acceptance of facial disfigurement are also important. This can take place in the form of teaching in schools and in the workplace. Teachers' expectations of pupils' academic achievements have been shown to be influenced by physical appearance, the more attractive children being regarded as more intelligent (Dion et al., 1972). This reinforces the need for education by those professionals involved in the care of this group of children.

Facial disfigurement is a constant and continuing source of disadvantage and stress for children and families. Some children will show remarkable resilience in coping with the situation but many will have a degree of impairment in their psychosocial functioning and development. Adults may choose a form of work where they have minimal contact with the general public; children are given fewer opportunities to show their real abilities (Hirst and Middleton, 1997).

There remains much to be done in educating society. There is also a need to increase professional health workers' awareness and understanding of the difficulties encountered and how to meet them. If professionals have difficulties in understanding the nature of visible differences, what hope is there that the general public can understand? Barriers can also be constructed by those with visible differences themselves, whose assumptions are based on previous experiences where society has rejected them.

Support groups are one way to help with the situation. Most groups have quite a local focus and are not resourced to cover a large provision of activities. However, regular closed group meetings, information giving, networking, emotional support, advocacy, therapeutic activities, lobbying and campaigning, educational work and research are among the many, varied opportunities provided. Groups may be run by professionals with an interest in the field, or by the families of children with disabilities, and by former patients. The diversity of members can both help and hinder the effectiveness of the group and the choice regarding membership must be based on a clear assessment of what the group can offer each individual member. National organizations exist alongside local self-help groups, attempting to meet the needs of their individual members. Self-help and support groups play a valuable role for individual members and can also be used as a force for change, functioning as a pressure group in increasing accountability, quality of care and resource availability. These groups provide a vital link between the hospital services and the often variable social services, providing a service that would otherwise be unavailable.

### The future

Imaging studies and surgical techniques continue to improve the cosmetic outcome for children with craniosynostosis. Many fundamental findings have been made through the genetic analysis of human syndromes in which craniosynostosis develops (Lajeunie et al., 1999). Further studies are required to construct the cascade of events that lead to osteoblast differentiation, and perhaps to propose treatment that might prevent the formation of craniosynostosis.

## A family's view

Claire was born with Crouzon's syndrome and also has hydrocephalus, which is treated with a shunt. She is now 20 years old and is considering becoming a doctor.

### Mum's view

Claire was the second child, born to healthy parents. She was born by Caesarean section and when Caroline, her mother, came round from the anaesthetic she found she had been placed in a room on her own. She was told the baby had been born with certain 'problems'. She didn't mind this and merely wanted to see Claire. She developed a particularly fierce desire to protect and support her baby.

The neurosurgeon examined Claire a few days later and diagnosed craniosynostosis. Being the daughter of a surgeon herself, Caroline examined various textbooks to establish whether her baby had a syndrome. The neurosurgeon felt it unhelpful to 'label' Claire so early, a decision that Caroline supported and from which she still feels she benefited. The diagnosis of Crouzon's syndrome came much later.

Caroline felt that the attitude of the neurosurgeon and the nursing staff was supportive and kind. She felt she could trust these professionals and could concentrate on looking after her baby herself, with their assistance.

Adrian, Claire's brother, paved the way for his little sister as she progressed through infant, primary and secondary school. The schools were chosen because they were co-educational and both children could attend. Adrian was always very caring and the two children remain very close in their adult life. Caroline feels there was never any question of treating Claire any differently from other children, although she did speak to the teachers and others, prior to starting each school. Caroline admits to 'bouts of nerves' when Claire went on a skiing trip and, later, when she went horseriding (she admits to feeling relieved when Claire gave the latter up).

Caroline has always been more concerned with the neurosurgical operations (shunt revisions) than the plastic surgery procedures, even though the last one (Le Fort III) was so extensive. This last procedure was discussed between Claire and both her parents. There was no doubt that it would be the correct treatment for Claire, but it was important that everyone felt it was the correct decision.

Caroline has always been impressed by the quality of nursing care: 'the sensitivity, gentle handling, understanding and professional knowledge are superb'. She also recognizes the importance of the developing role of the play specialist, which she views as complementary to patient care. She feels that the play specialists help the patient to counteract preconceptions and worries and to divert attention away from the more unpleasant or frightening procedures.

With regards to Crouzon's syndrome, Caroline admits her feelings and observations about this group of children are many and complex; and that they are often bright and lively youngsters who seem to give more to life than they take.

Finally, now that Claire has had most of her surgery, Caroline finds it 'remarkable to see the change not only in Claire's appearance, but also in the reactions of other people, both the general public and friends and relations. Everyone close to Claire has been very positive, and I tell her that I think she has crossed the boundary between looking different, and the rest of humanity.'

### Claire's view

As a child I always knew that I looked different to other children, but this never bothered me since I had not been brought up to think that I was different and I had been born that way, so it was all I knew . . . of course there was the situation of being stared at and being called names; the latter bothered me most when I was very young, and the former as I grew a little older. There were, however, ways in which I learned to deal with it such as ignoring the children or talking calmly. As I got older, I found that it was sometimes more useful to tell the teacher or my parents, whichever was relevant or necessary.

I never knew what the condition was or what it was called until I was in secondary school. This is probably because it never meant that much to me. It was just annoying at age 11 to be asked by my fellow pupils what had happened to me and not to have a specific answer other than calmly saying that I was born like this, and smiling, despite my annoyance at their rudeness.

One of Claire's earliest memories of hospital was of being taken by a nurse into a room full of people. She was about four or five at the time. These people came from all over the world and spoke very quietly and calmly. Claire felt terribly proud that all these people were so interested in her and she found the whole experience rather exciting; she feels it could only have added to her being so outgoing.

Claire describes the next 'major' thing that happened to her was when her shunt caused problems. She was 15 at the time and felt 'strange and dizzy'. She required several neurosurgical operations over the next 18 months including a period on external ventricular drainage due to a CSF infection.

Claire describes the nurses in the following way: 'They all knew what was happening and why I felt a certain way. They were also very comforting, sympathetic and patient with me, despite the fact that I felt awful, was constantly vomiting and drifted in and out of sleep a lot of the time.'

Claire also has memories of a CT scan, where she describes herself as not being aware of what was happening, but hearing 'quiet, comforting and reassuring voices that were not my parents'.

A series of craniofacial operations were later performed and Claire describes the fear of not being able to see her surroundings following her surgery (due to periorbital oedema) and of her total reliance on others. She describes the importance of people introducing themselves on entering her room, and of doctors and nurses explaining procedures before touching her. She describes the strangeness of nasal stents, nasogastric tubes and feeding, and how dreadful it was when these tubes were removed. She describes her frustration at not being understood in the initial days following her Le Fort III, because of the temporary difficulty with speech due to the dental and palatal surgery. She describes vivid memories of the nurses: 'The nurses took time out to talk to me, before the operation, during and after my worst days, to allay my worries and fears and any concerns I had, which I greatly appreciated.'

Claire recognizes the difficulties faced by parents during this time: 'I feel it is sometimes even worse for parents and relatives than it is for the patient.' She recognizes the value in parents being given 'time out' and being encouraged to leave the ward, with the confidence that their child will be well cared for in their absence.

Claire is pleased with her new appearance and feels that surgery was worth it; she feels more confident in herself.

# References

Barden RC, Ford ME, Jenson AG (1989) Effects of craniofacial disfigurement in infancy on the quality of mother–infant interactions. Child Development 60: 819–24.

Blank CE (1960). Apert's syndrome (a type of acrocephalosyndactyly) – observations on a British series of 39 cases. Annual of Human Genetics 24: 151–63.

Bradley E (1997) Understanding the problems. In Lansdowne R, Rumsey N, Bradbury E, Carr T, Partridge J (eds) Visibly Different. Coping with Disfigurement. Oxford: Butterworth-Heinemann, pp. 189–90.

Burton L (1975). The Family Life of Sick Children. London: Routledge & Kegan Paul.

Crittenden PM, Ainsworth MDS (1989) Child maltreatment and attachment theory. In Cichetti D, Carlson V (eds) Child Maltreatment: Theory and Research on the Causes and Consequences of Child Abuse and Neglect. Cambridge: Cambridge University Press, pp. 432–63.

Dion KK, Berschield E, Walster E (1972) What is beautiful is good. Journal of Personal Social Psychology 24: 285–90.

Gonzales S, Thompson D, Hayward R, Lane R (1996) Treatment of obstructive sleep apnoea using nasal CPAP in children with craniofacial dysostosis. Child's Nervous System 12: 713–9.

Hirst D, Middleton J (1997) Psychological intervention and models of current working practice. In Lansdowne L, Rumsey N, Bradbury E, Carr T, Partridge J (eds) Visibly Different. Coping with Disfigurement. Oxford: Butterworth-Heinemann, pp. 169–70.

Jennet B, Lindsay K (1994) Hydrocephalus and other cranial abnormalities. In An Introduction to Neurosurgery. Oxford: Butterworth-Heinemann, pp. 288–9.

Lajeunie E, Catala M, Renier D (1999) Craniosynostosis: from a clinical description to an understanding of bone formation of the skull. Child's Nervous System 15: 676–80.

Langios JH, Sawin DB (1981) Infant physical attractiveness as an elicitor of parenting behaviour. Paper presented at The Society for Research in Child Development, Boston.

Manger G (1983) Craniofacial surgery nursing: an overview. Canadian Nurse 4: 18–22.

May L (1992) Craniosynostosis – corrective surgery for a cosmetic defect. Professional Nurse (December) 176–8.

Thompson D, Harkness W, Jones B, Gonzales S, Andar U, Hayward R (1995) Subdural intracranial pressure monitoring in craniosynostosis: its surgical role. Child's Nervous System 11: 269–75.

Thompson D, Jones B, Hayward R, Harkness W (1994) Assessment and treatment of craniosynostosis. British Journal of Hospital Medicine 52(1): 17–24.

Virchow R (1851) Über den Cretinismus, namentlich in franken, und pathologische Schädelformen. Ver Phys Med Gesellsh Wurzburg 2: 230–71.

# Chapter 8
# Congenital malformations

## Anencephaly

The brain is represented by a dysfunctional mass of nervous tissue, which includes the primitive brain stem and a few cranial nerves. Failure of the neural groove to form into a tube, or gain a covering of mesoderm or ectoderm, results in exposure of the brain and its ultimate degeneration. Most of these foetuses are stillborn, but some may occasionally survive for a few hours.

## Encephalocoeles

The cranial equivalent of spina bifida is known as an encephalocoele. This rare condition occurs with an incidence between 0.1 and 0.5 per 1,000 live births (Martinez-Lage et al., 1996) and occurs most frequently in the occipital position, although anterior encephalocoeles do occur. The aetiology of encephalocoeles is unknown, although various environmental and genetic associations have been implicated (Peter and Fieggen, 1999).

Encephalocoeles may be associated with other abnormalities of the central nervous system, some of which may be secondary to the encephalocoele; such anomalies include craniosynostosis, oral clefting, absence of the corpus callosum, Dandy Walker Syndrome and Arnold Chiari malformations.

### Posterior encephalocoeles

Posterior encephalocoeles protrude through the occipital bone and occasionally through the foramen magnum and the atlas. Diagnosis is obvious at birth and the condition is usually compatible with life. The soft swelling protrudes through the underlying bone defect and may contain meninges alone, or meninges accompanied by cerebral tissue; this tissue may be functional but this is unlikely in small encephalocoeles. Indeed, small posterior encephaloceles may be of cosmetic significance only, although they may be a pointer to abnormalities underneath. Posterior encephalocoeles may be associated with other congenital abnormalities such as the Chiari type malformations, and hydrocephalus is a possibility. The head size is usually quite small.

## Clinical evaluation

Investigations include a plain X-ray to decipher the degree of underlying bone defect, and a CT or MRI scan to demonstrate the amount of cerebral tissue within the sac, and the presence of hydrocephalus.

Neurological examination at birth is often normal due to the immaturity of the brain, with such deficits as focal weaknesses, seizures, visual impairment, spasticity and cranial nerve involvement, becoming more obvious as the child develops.

Skin closure is usually complete, but there may be ulceration, weeping and infection. Careful handling and positioning of the encephalocoele is required, particularly in those cases where hydrocephalus may result in a rapid increase in size of the sac.

Antenatal screening may have prepared the family, but encouragement may be required to help the mother bond with her baby, and practical advice given when handling her child. Race, religion and cultural background may affect the parents' attitude to their baby, and various members of the multidisciplinary team including the social worker will be involved.

## Preoperative assessment

Discussions with the parents concerning the ethics of surgery are important. These lesions will enlarge due to herniation of the brain and the presence of hydrocephalus, they are unsightly and present significant nursing problems; they may become necrotic and occasionally rupture, leading to meningitis. Surgical excision is therefore recommended except in cases where the baby's condition is clearly not compatible with life. The surgeon must ensure that the parents are aware of the risks of surgery with regard to mortality and morbidity. There must also be a clear understanding that, although surgery is aimed at preserving existing neurological function, it is unlikely to improve it.

In addition to the usual care requirements of the neonate, these infants may require feeding via a nasogastric tube, and attention must be given to temperature control due to excessive heat loss from the head. The usual blood profile will be necessary and adequate blood cross matched.

# Surgery

Most encephalocoeles are skin covered, so a delayed approach to surgery may be considered. For those babies with exposed neural tissue or CSF leakage, surgery should be undertaken as an emergency. Surgery is aimed at preserving normal cerebral tissue where possible and replacement or excision of dysplastic brain tissue; the sac will be removed and a watertight repair performed; treatment of hydrocephalus may be undertaken during this initial surgery, or reassessed at a later date where necessary; further cosmetic repair may occasionally be required at a later date.

# Postoperative care

The needs of these babies following surgery involve the normal requirements of a small baby; warmth, nutrition and comfort are all essential, and the mother can be encouraged to provide these now that her baby is easier to handle. She may feel more confident in her own abilities, and in her child's appearance and 'acceptability'. The multidisciplinary team should be aware of the emotions the parents may be feeling, and provide support and encouragement to them.

As previously mentioned, hydrocephalus may occur and, if it is not treated during the initial operation, may necessitate monitoring and future treatment.

# Discharge

Should the baby's recovery be uneventful and feeding be established, it may be discharged from hospital. The baby's immediate needs may be those of a normal baby, although the family may require much support from the community team in coming to terms with what the future may bring. As the baby grows and develops, so his needs will become more apparent and, with this, the appropriate care requirements will become evident. Each child is individual, and the outcome variable and unpredictable.

# Outlook

There is a 9% to 47% mortality rate during the first few years of life for those children born with an occipital encephalocoele (Date et al., 1993). A poor prognosis is associated with the amount of neuronal tissue in the sac, microcephaly, and the presence of hydrocephalus; poor vision, developmental delay, incontinence and poor motor function may occur. An improved outcome has been found to be associated with a normal head size at birth, a normal neurological assessment, the absence of migrational disorders, and hydrocephalus (Martinez-Lage et al., 1996). Timing of surgery does not appear to relate to the long-term outcome.

## Anterior encephalocoeles

Most anterior encephalocoeles are apparent at birth, with a skin-covered swelling in the midline, and hypertelorism. This may not have been anticipated by antenatal screening, and consequently parents may shocked and distressed by their baby's appearance. Explanation and reassurance should be given, and time should be allowed for discussion and adjustment. The outlook for the majority of these babies in terms of development is good, although this may need to be reiterated to parents as they try to adjust to a baby who looks abnormal.

The requirements for this rare group of babies are similar to those described above. However, because handling is easier due to the position of the encephalocoele, and the outlook brighter, bonding between mother and child is usually easier.

Following an MRI scan, surgical excision will be undertaken via a bifrontal approach. The majority of frontal encephalocoeles contain gliotic, non-functional cerebral tissue that can be divided from the normal brain and the skin cosmetically repaired. Mild hypertelorism can be corrected in early childhood, but a more severe defect may need orbital repositioning at a later stage. Hydrocephalus may develop in 10% to 20% of children with anterior lesions (Simpson et al., 1984). Unless associated with other central nervous system abnormalities or syndromic disorders, 60% to 85% of children born with frontal encephalocoeles will be of normal intelligence and have normal motor skills (MacFarlane et al., 1995).

Frontonasal masses, transsphenoidal encephalocoeles and nasal gliomas are often first encountered by the ENT team, when the baby has presented with nasopharyngeal obstruction. Surgery will usually involve the ENT surgeon and neurosurgeon together. In the case of a nasal glioma there may be no skull defect and surgery may reveal merely an intracranial fibrous connection. The outcome for this group of children should be favourable in terms of mortality and morbidity.

## Basal encephalocoeles

These are extremely rare, and protrude through defects in the basal skull bones. They may contain hypothalamic, chiasmal and pituitary structures. Temporal lobe epilepsy and occasionally CSF leaks due to fistulas of the ear or nose with recurrent meningitis may be the first indication of the presence of a basal encephalocoele. The outcome is related to the structures involved and the degree of that involvement. Basal encephalocoeles, but particularly transsphenoidal lesions, carry a mortality rate of 50% and long-term endocrinological handicap rate of 70% (Kennedy et al., 1997).

## The future

The outcome factors described for those babies with occipital encephalocoeles apply to all children with encephalocoeles. The association of other serious CNS anomalies is also a major factor in predicting poor neurological outcome, but hydrocephalus is only a negative factor if present at birth (Fenstermaker et al., 1984).

Further research is necessary into the disordered embryogenesis of congenital brain anomalies, and into the aetiology behind such devastating abnormalities as encephalocoeles.

## Arachnoid cysts and the Dandy Walker complex

Abnormal development of the arachnoid membrane is one of the causes of an intracranial arachnoid cyst, although such cysts can occur due to local arachnoiditis following trauma, or brain atrophy. Arachnoid cysts exist within the subarachnoid space and are filled with CSF. The deficits within the walls of the cyst restrict the outward flow of CSF and so the cyst enlarges.

### Clinical evaluation

The signs and symptoms may be related to the site of the cyst, but are more usually due to hydrocephalus or raised intracranial pressure. Presentation is often delayed, being discovered only when the child is being investigated for headache, seizures or learning difficulties.

Routine antenatal screening with ultrasound may detect a significant number of children with unexpected cystic abnormalities, and the surgical management of these children remains controversial. Computerized tomography and MRI scanning will make the diagnosis of arachnoid cysts for those children presenting later in life fairly straightforward, although haemorrhage and infection will complicate the interpretation. Hydrocephalus is seen commonly with suprasellar and posterior fossa cysts.

### Surgery

Arachnoid cysts causing mass effects or hydrocephalus require surgery (Wang et al., 1998). However, complete surgical removal of the cyst is rare due to the attachment of much of the wall of the cyst to the surrounding brain. Surgery, therefore, is aimed at reducing the volume of the cyst by endoscopic fenestration or insertion of a shunt.

### Outcome

The co-operative European study showed that only 18% of cysts completely disappeared whatever the surgical choice (Oberbauer et al., 1992). A favourable outcome is associated with a significant reduction in cyst size, but the site of the cyst is also significant, with suprasellar cysts having a high failure rate and temporal lobe cysts having the best (Richard et al., 1989).

Cognitive outcome is generally favourable, but is dependent on the location and size of the cyst, and success of surgery.

### Dandy Walker malformation

This condition comprises a cystic enlargement of the fourth ventricle, with foraminal atresia and atrophy of the surrounding brain. It causes hydrocephalus and may be associated with other abnormalities such as agenesis of the corpus callosum and Arnold Chiari malformation. Treatment consists of insertion of a shunt for hydrocephalus, or occasionally direct shunting of the cyst itself. It seems that treatment of the cyst itself does not enhance cerebellar function (Gerszten and Albright, 1995) and morbidity remains high despite surgical treatment, with subnormal intelligence and learning disabilities occurring in as many as 71% of cases (Sawaya and McLaurin, 1981).

### The future

Neuroendoscopic treatment of arachnoid cysts may well be the way forward but will only partially alleviate the difficulties faced by these children and their families. Real progress must be through a greater understanding of the neurobiology involved in the formation of intracerebral cysts, which will allow effective prevention strategies.

The Nobel Laureate Oe (Oe, 1982) provides a moving illustration for the dedication and creativity of the human spirit when faced with a child born with an encephalocoele, but for the majority of families, sadness and difficulties prevail. As healthcare providers, we must support their individual physical and emotional needs.

## Arnold Chiari malformation

This describes a spectrum of abnormalities of increasing severity and mainly involves the hind brain. There are four types of Chiari malformation, types one and two being the most common. The embryogenesis remains controversial.

Chiari type I consists of elongated, peg-like cerebellar tonsils, which protrude through the foramen magnum. Parts of the fourth ventricle may also herniate downwards. Hydrocephalus rarely occurs and symptoms are due to compression of the brain stem at the foramen magnum. It is often associated with syringomyelia and may not be diagnosed until adolescence or early adulthood, when pain is the principal symptom. Treatment is only indicated at this point, when pain and progressive motor impairment are evident. Treatment consists of insertion of a shunt for hydrocephalus if indicated, and cervical medullary decompression.

Chiari type II is present in most children with spina bifida, and is responsible for the development of hydrocephalus in these children. There is downward displacement of the vermis, the brain stem, the cerebellar tonsils and the fourth ventricle, through into the upper parts of the cervical canal. Compression of the brain stem can result in abnormalities affecting all associated functions, and obstruction to the outflow of CSF from the fourth ventricle leads to hydrocephalus. Syringomyelia can also occur as the CSF is forced downwards from the fourth ventricle into the central canal of the spinal cord, causing dilation. A shunt may be fitted to relieve hydrocephalus. Occasionally, a decompression craniectomy may be necessary, involving decompression of the posterior fossa, foramen magnum and upper cervical canal; the aim of this surgery is to leave the brain in its abnormal position, while allowing it the opportunity for maximum recovery and potential. The outcome from surgery is variable due to the existing brain constriction from thickened adherent arachnoid and bony surroundings.

Chiari type III is a rare and complex malformation, involving an occipital cervical encephalocoele, which encloses the prolapsed cerebellar tissue. It is sometimes associated with Klipper-Feil syndrome (which involves a short neck, limited neck motion and an abnormally low hairline posteriorly). Despite successful treatment of the hydrocephalus and the encephalocoele itself, severe developmental delay occurs. Aggressive treatment is indicated to ease the care of the child and to offer the maximum potential.

Chiari type IV describes a hypoplasia of the cerebellar hemisphere. There is no recommended intervention and treatment is aimed at symptom management.

## A family's view

Kim was born following a normal pregnancy and delivery, with a small occipital encephalocoele. This was removed in the neonatal period and

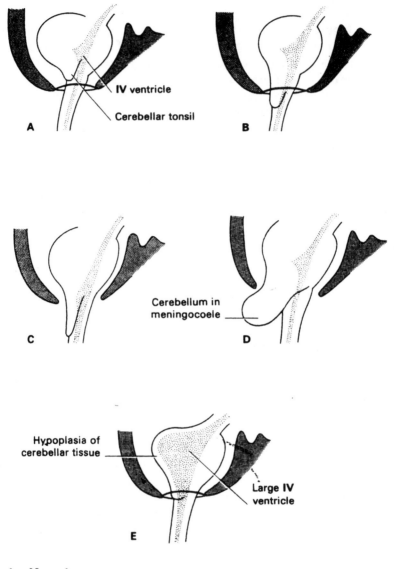

A    Normal.
B    Chiari type I.
C    Chiari type II (Arnold Chiari).
D    Chiari type III.
E    Chiari type IV.

**Figure 8.1.** Arnold Chiari malformations (reprinted from Haywood R (1980) Essentials of Neurosurgery, with permission of Blackwell Science Ltd, Oxford).

she also required a shunt insertion for hydrocephalus. She required numerous shunt revisions during her first few years of life. Although able to walk, Kim became increasingly ataxic during adolescence. It was discovered that she had developed syringomyelia and a foramen magnum decompression was performed whereby approximately 4 cm of suboccipital bone around the foramen magnum was removed, thus providing a decompression; Kim's walking improved a little following this, but she remains ataxic.

Kim is deaf and has global developmental delay.

## Mum's view

I had my 21st birthday just after Kim was born; nothing could have prepared me for what lay ahead. I was surprised when Kim was born with this lump on the back of her head and the doctors did tell both of us that she might have quite a few problems, but they didn't know what they'd be, or how badly she might be affected. So we just got on with it. The shunt was a pain, always going wrong, why couldn't they get it right?

When we realized Kim was deaf, I learnt the Makaton sign language so I could communicate with her; she never really progressed onto adult signing, so we realized that her learning was slow. Her walking came late, but she did seem to be able to get around OK.

Kim attended a school for the deaf and, although her progress was slow, she remained a cheerful and loving child. As the family expanded, Kim was very much part of the family unit. Life was difficult though. Kim's developmental delay became more obvious as she got older.

It's like she just never grew up. The problems with her walking were tough and, after the decompression surgery, things improved a bit, but she remains unsteady. She's 17 now and we had to have her care transferred to adult hospital. That was awful for us and her, like a security blanket being taken away. We went to an outpatient's appointment and Kim was agitated and upset; the doctor was OK, but he didn't know Kim or what she'd been through, he seemed a bit busy for us. Not a brilliant start.

I'm scared of what will happen in the future, when we're too old to care for Kim. We do have lots of help and support, and we do use the respite place occasionally, but we don't want Kim to be put away.

## Kim's view

When in hospital, Kim always expressed (through Makaton) that she wanted to go home! As she got older, mum would not always be resident with her in hospital as she had small children at home, and Kim would be reasonably content as long as there was a consistent nurse caring for her. Communication was a problem, even with signing boards, and Kim was frustrated and frightened at times. She was a friendly and affectionate child, and Mum said that, although she hated being in hospital, she quite liked all the attention, especially from the 'play lady'.

As she has grown up, Kim has continued to depend heavily on her parents, but has made friends and maintained relationships with her school friends. She appears to enjoy life.

She still wants to go back to her 'old' hospital!

# References

Date L, Yagyu Y, Asari S, Ohmoto T (1993) Long-term outcome in surgically treated encephaloceles. Surgical Neurology 40: 125–30.

Fenstermaker RA, Roessmann U, Rekate HL (1984) Fourth ventriculoceles with extracranial extension. Journal of Neurosurgery 61: 348–50.

Gerszten PC, Albright AL (1995) Relationship between cerebellar appearance and function in children with Dandy Walker Syndrome. Pediatric Neurosurgery. 23: 86–92.

Kennedy EM, Gruber DP, Bilmore DA, Crone KR (1997) Transpalatal approach for the extracranial surgical repair of transsphenoidal encephaloceles in children. Journal of Neurosurgery 87: 677–81.

MacFarlane R, Rutka JT, Armstrong D, Philips J, Posnick J, Forte V, Humphries RP, Drake J, Hoffman HJ (1995) Encephaloceles of the anterior cranial fossa, management and outcome. Pediatric Neurosurgery 23: 148–58.

Martinez-Lage JF, Pusa M, Sola J, Soler CL, Montalvo CG, Domingo R, Puche A, Roman FH, Asorin P, Lasso R (1996) The child with an encephalocele: etiology, neuroimaging and outcome. Child's Nervous System 12: 540–50.

Oberbauer RW, Hasse J, Pucher R (1992) Arachnoid cysts in children: a European co-operative study. Child's Nervous System 8: 281–6.

Oe K (1982 ) A Personal Matter. (Trans. J Nathan.) New York: Grove Weidenfield (Evergreen End).

Peter J, Fieggen G (1999) Congenital malformations of the brain – a neurosurgical perspective at the close of the twentieth century. Child's Nervous System 15: 635–45.

Richard KE, Dahl K, Sanker P (1989) Long-term follow up of children and juveniles with arachnoid cysts. Child's Nervous System 5: 184–7.

Sawaya R, McLaurin RL (1981) Dandy-Walker syndrome. Clinical analysis of 23 cases. Journal of Neurosurgery 55: 89–98.

Simpson BA, David JI, White J (1984) Cephaloceles: treatment, outcome and antenatal diagnosis. Neurosurgery 15: 14–21.

Wang TJ, Lin HC, Lui HM, Tseng CL, Shen YZ (1998) Intracranial arachnoid cysts in children: related signs and associated anomalies. Pediatric Neurology 19: 100–4.

# Chapter 9
# Paediatric vascular disorders

Cerebrovascular malformations are developmental in nature and result from failure of the embryonic vascular network. Many lesions are asymptomatic and only found incidentally or at autopsy, so the incidence of these malformations is unclear. They are, however, rare in children, and most clinical research is adult based. There are four major categories: telangiectases, which are capillary lesions of little clinical significance; venous malformations, composed of anomalous veins that drain into a dilated venous trunk, which may cause seizures and haemorrhage and consequently require surgery; cavernous haemangiomas, which are low-flow, purple, nodular lesions, often calcified, may cause seizures and haemorrhage, and thus require surgery; and arteriovenous malformations (AVMs).

## Arteriovenous malformations

An arteriovenous malformation is the most common cerebrovascular lesion that causes symptoms in children. However, the most common age of presentation is between 20 and 40 years, which would suggest a change in the malformation's evolution. The majority of the cerebral vascular tree is formed by 60 days' gestation so one would assume that any malformation would become symptomatic before the patient reached 20 years of age. There must therefore be delayed factors that influence the development and declaration of the AVM (Humphreys, 1999).

An AVM consists of a mass of abnormal, dilated blood vessels that shunt arterial blood into the venous system without the normal connecting capillary network. The result is an elevated blood supply at high pressure, running through the abnormally fragile vessels of the AVM. Haemorrhage, ischaemia and stroke can occur.

### Clinical presentation

Arteriovenous malformations vary in clinical presentation according to their position and the age of the child. A greater number of children compared with adults experience haemorrhage as the first symptom. Haemorrhage occurs in 50% to 80% of children with AVM and it carries an average mortality rate of 15% and an average serious morbidity rate of 30% (Fults and Kelly, 1984). The risk of rehaemorrhaging in children treated conservatively is unknown due to the lack of data.

Progressive neurological deficits occur more commonly in adults, and this is attributed to ischaemia resulting from vascular 'steal'. Hydrocephalus may occur due to ventricular compression from dilated veins; headaches can also occur and, occasionally, seizures.

## Investigations

A CT scan will demonstrate cerebral haemorrhage after a ruptured AVM. Although an MRI scan will give better information, the explosive nature of the child's presentation, with sudden onset of severe headache and a deteriorating level of consciousness, will often not allow the time required for an MRI.

In the elective situation, both MRI scanning and angiography will be undertaken. Even in those children with an intracerebral haemorrhage small enough to be treated conservatively, angiography should be performed at presentation and at follow up: they may harbour a more occult malformation than their presentation suggests.

## Treatment

Treatment is aimed at achieving a complete cure of the malformation where possible, and this may be in the form of a surgical excision, or embolization. Four-fifths of children who haemorrhage from an AVM will need surgery to remove the blood clot and AVM, and to preserve the child's neurology (Humphreys, 1999).

Total surgical excision may be possible, depending on the size and location of the AVM, and occasionally surgery will be necessary in two stages. Haemorrhage during surgery from the AVM itself is less likely than in the case of an aneurysm; however, the operation may be prolonged due to the necessity of removing both the clot and the AVM, and this can increase the risk factor for the very small child.

The role of endovascular treatment in the management of these children has gradually increased over the past decade. However, the majority of AVMs in children are small, with vessels that are difficult to cannulate, even with today's microcatheters. Partial obliteration of the AVM may alleviate some of the symptoms, but there is no evidence that it will protect against haemorrhage.

Radiosurgery has seldom been used in the treatment of AVMs in children, but in those cases where the gamma knife has been used, there are early encouraging results in carefully selected patients (Altschuler et al., 1989). This may, however, be attributed to the less invasive approach to the lesion and the reduction in hospitalization.

### Preoperative care

Where the child's condition allows, surgery should be delayed and performed as an elective procedure. If surgery can be delayed for a week following haemorrhage, the brain will be more relaxed and the haematoma partially liquefied. Cerebral vasospasm seldom occurs in children, but rebleeding can occur. Thus careful observation of the child is required with regard to neurological status. Bed rest, a darkened environment and analgesia are recommended; stool softeners should be given to avoid straining during defecation. Parents can be encouraged to help in their child's care by working alongside the nurse, providing safety, hygiene, and a quiet and calm environment.

It remains debatable whether obliteration of the malformation itself influences neurological outcome in terms of development, seizure activity or headaches (Troupp, 1976) and research continues in this area. However, the risk of rebleeding is such that treatment is advocated in the majority of cases.

### Postoperative care

Postoperative care will be similar to that required for a craniotomy for tumour removal (see Chapter 4), with additional consideration given to the possibility of rebleeding should the initial removal of the AVM be incomplete. In this case, the surgeon may request that the child continues to be on bed rest in a quiet environment until definitive surgery is undertaken.

The child's rehabilitation needs must be assessed individually and based on the degree of cerebellar, motor and speech deficits involved. Prophylactic anticonvulsants will usually be continued for up to two years following surgery, although for those children who presented with a large parenchymal haemorrhage, chronic epilepsy may necessitate long-term anticonvulsant medication.

# Cavernous haemangiomas

A cavernoma is classified as a hamartoma, and can occur outside the CNS, including the musculoskeletal system, the liver, kidney and skin. The incidence of cavernous haemangiomas can be sporadic or familial (autosomal dominant), may occur as single or multiple lesions, and can increase or reduce in size.

Intracerebrally, these purple lobulated malformations occur most frequently in the cerebral hemispheres. Macroscopically, they resemble a honeycomb, with irregular vascular spaces of varying sizes. The structure of the walls of these vascular spaces makes them susceptible to rupture and blood flow inside the lesion is slow with a correspondingly high rate of thrombosis.

The intracerebral lesion can be totally asymptomatic or can produce symptoms including seizures, increasing neurological deficit, and haemorrhage.

Diagnosis is by CT and MRI scan, angiography providing information in some cases.

Treatment consists of surgical excision in those children who are symptomatic, although the long-term outcome depends on the location of the cavernoma and any existing neurological deficit. Radiotherapy has shown to be ineffective.

## Spinal arteriovenous fistulas and malformations

These occur rarely in childhood. They are often asymptomatic, discovered on routine examination and confirmed on MRI scanning. The management of these fistulas must involve a very low level of risk in view of the unknown natural history of the disease. Although a combined approach can be considered when managing these children, endovascular treatment has become the way forward, despite the fact that a complete cure cannot always be achieved.

## Cerebral aneurysms

The incidence of multiple aneurysms is lower in children than in adults, but giant aneurysms occur most frequently in children. There is no evidence to suggest that aneurysms are congenital in nature, and aneurysms in children appear to be related to a vessel wall matrix weakening process, rather than being caused by such haemodynamic factors as shear stress (teBrugge, 1999). Since the number of aneurysms diagnosed is highest between the ages of 35 to 60 years, the theory of a degenerative vascular disease process is a likely factor in adulthood.

Most patients are asymptomatic until the time of aneurysm rupture, when blood is forced into the subarachnoid space resulting in a subarachnoid haemorrhage (SAH). Seventy per cent of survivors will suffer a major disability following SAH (Herrick and Gelb, 1992), and the risk of rebleeding is high. Care is aimed at controlling blood pressure and vasospasm (the latter occurrence being rare in children), providing analgesia, and ensuring a quiet and calm environment. Surgery is the main treatment following diagnosis by CT and MRI scanning, and angiography. The outcome is very variable, and largely depends on the degree of haemorrhage and the area of brain involved.

Endovascular treatment is producing good outcomes, although a combined approached may be required in the management of giant aneurysms.

## Aneurysm of the vein of Galen

There are two variations of this rare paediatric vascular lesion, but both involve a vast arterial supply. Located within the subarachnoid space, vein of Galen aneurysms can be diagnosed prenatally.

Neonates presenting with vein of Galen malformation will usually have secondary congestive cardiac failure and initially will be managed conservatively; occasionally, transarterial embolization has been attempted to bring these children into a haemodynamically stable state, but this remains a technically difficult procedure. The majority of children with vein of Galen malformations present later on, during the first year of life, with an increasing head circumference and hydrocephalus. Periodic developmental assessment and imaging are essential in deciding the appropriate time for intervention; the therapeutic window for optimal endovascular management is between four and six months of age (teBrugge, 1999). The goal of treatment is to reduce venous pressure by diminishing the arteriovenous shunt and allowing normal CSF hydrodynamics to develop. Surgical shunting is now discouraged as it is associated with a reduced morbidity. Positive outcomes for these children are now being reported if endovascular treatment is given during the therapeutic window and this must be assessed for each individual child (Lasjaunias and Alvarez, 1996). However, it may be necessary to stage the embolization procedures, with as many as three separate episodes being undertaken during the child's first two years of life if the aneurysm or the child's status is not amenable to a single procedure.

### Outcome

Despite anatomical cure being achieved for many of these babies after embolization, their neurological condition is rarely reported. Those studies that have been published regarding transvenous approaches describe a high proportion of deaths or disabled children (Ciricillo et al.,

1990). However, as techniques continue to be refined and there is a greater understanding of the hydrovenous state of the child and the relevance of this to the outcome, improved results are being obtained: 66% of children are being reported as neurologically normal following transarterial embolization (a more technically difficult procedure than transvenous embolization), with an additional 14% reportedly neurologically normal with anticonvulsant medication (Berenstein and Lasjaunias, 1992).

## Childhood stroke

The causes of ischaemic stroke in childhood are varied, and in the majority of cases a specific aetiological cause can be found. These include trauma, metabolic disorders, cardiac disorders, infection and vasculopathies. Consequently, treatment is aimed at the underlying cause of the stroke and at providing brain protection. For those children presenting with ischaemic stroke in the future, intra-arterial or intravenous endovascular recanalization techniques will be proposed.

However, in specific cases such as Moyamoya disease, surgery is now performed. Moyamoya disease describes an unusual vascular lesion of unknown aetiology. There is progressive arterial narrowing or obstruction of major intracranial cerebral arteries; numerous collateral vessels develop at the base of the brain in an attempt to perfuse a brain that has been rendered ischaemic by occlusion of one or more vessels. Repeated ischaemic episodes may occur, along with haemorrhagic strokes due to the presence of abnormal blood vessels. Ischaemic symptoms usually develop from cerebral infarction and are associated with neurological deficits and intellectual impairement. Seizures are common.

The greatest incidence of Moyamoya disease is in Japan, although the precise genetics remain unclear. The disease peaks in the first decade of life, or in the fourth decade. An onset before six years of life, increasing severity of presenting deficits and severe disease demonstrated on angiography indicate a poor prognosis (Maki and Onomoto, 1988).

Attempts at revascularization to improve the brain's available collateral circulation have at times proved successful. There are two main types of revascularization, direct and indirect. Direct vascularization includes a procedure known as EC–IC bypass, where revascularization is attempted from the extracranial to the intracranial circulation; this procedure is cumbersome to perform in the small child and the risk of perioperative ischaemia is present. Some patients have shown clinical improvement a year later, with an improved collateral circulation (Matsushima et al., 1999). Indirect vascularization describes grafting of a muscle or artery onto the brain surface and hence generating blood vessel formation; revascularization from indirect bypass begins to develop two weeks after surgery and becomes well developed three months following surgery (Kinugasa et al., 1993).

For those children with Moyamoya disease, however, the benefit may be short lived, with ischaemic strokes continuing to occur in multiple areas. Very long-term prognosis is unknown, although the progression of the disease process itself involves the formation of Moyamoya vessels, and consequently would suggest a continuing clinical deterioration. Early diagnosis and surgical intervention, coupled with screening of those children thought be of high risk (those with a family history of Moyamoya disease) would improve prognosis for this group of children (Ishikawa et al., 1997).

## The future

Advances in biological knowledge coupled with advances in treatment options and strategies contribute to the therapeutic care and management of paediatric vascular malformations. Each child's individual requirements must be evaluated when coming to decisions regarding treatment options available. As with other rare childhood diseases, sharing of information and research is essential to ensure optimum outcomes.

## A family's view

Susan is a 15-year-old child and was admitted to her local hospital with a five-day history of headaches and a two-day history of vomiting, blurred vision, difficulty in hearing and general ataxia with a mild right hemiparesis. A CT scan was reported as showing an aneurysm and cerebral haemorrhage; she was transferred to a paediatric neurosurgical ward where an MRI scan showed a brainstem cavernous haemangioma. She was unable to walk by this time and had severe hearing loss. She was commenced on dexamethasone, a thorough assessment was undertaken, and a craniotomy was performed for total removal of the cavernoma. Her recovery was slow but steady and, on transfer back to her local hospital, she had a resolving right hemiporesis and general ataxia. She had a gaze palsy to the left, diplopia, nystagmus and decreased sensation of the left fifth and seventh cranial nerves, and she also had a mild right sensorineural hearing loss and severe left sensorineural and retrocochlear hearing loss. Despite this, Susan was positive and cheerful and her cognitive skills appeared unscathed.

Susan's paternal aunt had died at 32 years old from a 'cerebral blood clot', her grandfather at 48 from a 'brain clot' and her grandmother at 62, also from a 'brain clot'. In view of this family history, Susan and her parents were referred to a geneticist. Susan's mother had recently finished chemotherapy for cervical cancer.

### Mum's view

> We had seen the GP several times with Susan the week before we got admitted to hospital, and I'm angry about that, especially with all her dad's family history. I was terrified she was going to die before she got operated on, everything took so long. I know how long things take in hospital from my own treatment, so I knew why it was happening; my husband was very agitated.

Susan's mother was quite withdrawn initially and kept herself to herself, rarely asking questions. We tried to involve her in talking to Susan about what had happened and what was about to happen in terms of surgery. Her husband explained that she was quite run down following chemotherapy and was finding everything utterly exhausting as well as frightening. He talked a little to Susan about her condition and treatment.

Following surgery, Susan's parents were clearly delighted and her father, in particular, helped with her physiotherapy and frequently walked her up and down the corridor once her condition allowed. Susan vomited for days following surgery despite antiemetics, and Mum was empathetic with her daughter. Gradually Mum became more involved in Susan's care and rehabilitation, and became more responsive to her surroundings. She was clearly quite a private woman and had no wish to discuss sensitive issues with those around her. She did, however, express relief at her daughter's slow recovery, explaining that once surgery was over she realized that Susan's deficits were going to require hard work from herself as well as from Susan if things were to improve. She relied quite heavily on her husband but clearly had a good relationship with Susan, understanding and addressing her daughter's emotional needs.

Mum was keen to move back to her local hospital in terms of location, but needed reassurance from the team that Susan was in a safe condition for her to do so, and that she would receive appropriate care (she voiced concern about the lack of physiotherapy input she herself had received at the same hospital). Good communication with the team locally addressing Mum's specific concerns, and a referral to the local physiotherapist, did much to reassure her and make the transition back to the local hospital easier.

Mum said she 'couldn't believe the nightmare was over'. Her own diagnosis meant an ever-present possibility of recurrence and she had found it difficult to believe that Susan's illness could not also reoccur.

## Susan's view

I was really scared, I didn't know what was happening to me; I was scared of telling my Mum because she had all her own worries. When I could hardly walk or hear, I thought I might die like my relatives, I thought I must have cancer, like my Mum.

The scan was scary, and mum and dad were being odd. When I got transferred to the other hospital, there were all these really ill children and I thought I must be really ill too. They put me in a cubicle to start with and that was good, because I didn't have to see all those ill children. I had another scan and then a doctor told me why I couldn't walk or hear properly, and that I needed an operation. He told me he thought I would be OK, but that things might seem a bit worse after the operation; that was alright, at least I wasn't going to die and I didn't have cancer.

I felt really bad for ages after the operation. My head hurt and I was sick all the time, every time I moved. So I didn't move. But everyone kept nagging me and the physiotherapy was horrible. They kept giving me medicine into my drip but it didn't stop me throwing up. I think I slept a lot. I had an eye patch to stop me seeing double and that really helped but I'm glad none of my friends saw me, I'd have been so embarrassed.

Mum and Dad stayed with me the whole time, which was great, but I wish they'd left me alone sometimes. I wanted to watch telly, or sleep, and some of the nurses were quite cool and funny, but my Mum was always there, so I couldn't have a laugh with them. Sometimes they'd come and chat to me when Mum and Dad went out for a meal in the evening, and that was OK (depending who it was!). Some of them weren't much older than me; they're kind, but they do horrible things sometimes. Why does anyone want to be a nurse? The surgeon was OK. He came to see me most days in the morning, when I was still in bed, and he'd say 'not out of bed yet?' And I'd have had a really bad night throwing up and feeling awful; I think he thought he was being funny. But I'm glad the operation went OK – at least he said it did. There was a play lady, she gave me videos, painted my nails and talked to me. Most of the time I just wanted to sleep.

Everything is taking so long to get better, but I can walk better now and the eye patch helps me too. I want to go nearer home, but I don't want my school friends to laugh at me, so I asked mum to let my good friends come and see me, not anyone else. I'm very tired all the time, but the doctors say that will get better, that I've been very ill and have to take it easy (how can I take it easy with the physiotherapy, and my Dad wanting me to get up and walk all the time?). When I get home, he'll have to go back to work. I know he's trying to help me get better, but I'm OK now.

# References

Altschuler EM, Lunsford LD, Coffey RJ, Bissonette DJ, Flickinger JC (1989) Gamma knife surgery for intracranial arteriovenous malformations in childhood and adolescence. Pediatric Neuroscience 15: 53–61.

Berenstein A, Lasjaunias P (1992) Arteriovenous Fistulas of the Brain. (Surgical neuroangiography, Vol 4.) Berlin, Heidelberg, New York: Springer, pp. 267–317.

Ciricillo S, Edwards SM, Schmidt K, Hieshima G (1990) Interventional neuroradiological management of vein of Galen in neonates. Neurosurgery 27: 22–8.

Fults D, Kelly DL Jr (1984) Natural history of arteriovenous malformations of the brain: a clinical study. Neurosurgery 15: 658–62.

Herrick IA, Gelb AW (1992) Anesthesia for intracranial aneurysm surgery. Journal of Clinical Anesthesia 4: 73–82.

Humphreys R (1999) Brain vascular malformations. In Choux M, Di Rocco C, Hockley A, Walker M (eds) Pediatric Neurosurgery. London, Edinburgh, New York, Philadelphia, Sydney, Toronto: Churchill Livingstone, pp. 665–77.

Kinugasa K, Mandai S, Kamata I, Sugie K, Ohmoto T (1993) Surgical treatment of Moyamoya disease: operative technique for encephalo-duro-arterio-myo-synangiosis, its follow up, clinical results and angiograms. Neurosurgery 33: 527–31.

Ishikawa T, Kiyohiro H, Kamiyama H, Hiroshi Abe (1997) Effects of surgical revascularization on outcome of patients with Moya moya disease. Stroke 28(6): 1170–3.

Lasjaunias P, Alvarez A (1996) Aneurysmal malformations of the vein of Galen. Follow up of 120 children treated between 1984 and 1994. Interventional Radiology 2: 15–26.

Maki Y, Onomoto T (1988) Moyamoya disease. Child's Nervous System 4: 204–12.

Matsushima T, Inoue T, Suzuki So, Fujii K, Fukui M, Hasuo K (1999) Surgical treatment of Moyamoya disease in pediatric patients: comparison between the results of indirect and direct revascularization procedures. Neurosurgery 31: 401–5.

teBrugge K (1999) Neurointerventional procedures in the pediatric agegroup. Child's Nervous System 15: 751–54.

Troupp H (1976) Arteriovenous malformations of the brain. What are the indications for operation? In Morley TP (ed.) Current Controversies in Neurosurgery. Philadelphia PA: WB Saunders, pp. 212–16.

# Useful hints

## Hydrocephalus

- Children with shunts can swim and take part in sports. Rugby and other sports that may involve head contact, are discouraged.
- Travelling abroad and by aeroplane is feasible with a shunt; however, parents are recommended to take out a good medical insurance to cover any eventuality and to go to countries only where good paediatric services are available
- Vaccinations. Advice concerning vaccinations is variable and should be discussed between the parents and their paediatrician. However, the Association of Spina Bifida and Hydrocephalus (ASBAH) supplies an advice sheet regarding vaccination for children with shunts *in situ*. Generally speaking, hydrocephalus and the presence of a shunt are not reasons for withholding vaccination.
- A child with a shunt *in situ* may be tipped head down during play, physiotherapy and so forth; the valve system will prevent backflow of CSF up the shunt system.

## Brain tumours

- MRI scans can be performed when metal clips are still *in situ*. However, it is advisable to discuss this with the neuroradiologist prior to scanning.
- For those children who have problems with swallowing, the following may be useful. Place a teaspoon in the fridge prior to using – this facilitates easier mouth and swallowing actions; thicker fluids (such as yoghurts) are easier to control than water when swallowing; pureed or high water content products are recommended, given at frequent intervals.
- Healthcare workers have a responsibility to look after themselves and to take appropriate steps to manage stress. The National Association of

Staff Support (NASS) produces literature and holds conferences which help raise awareness of the need for support and how to implement this.

## Epilepsy

- Encourage a normal active life wherever possible.
- Encourage reintegration into peer group.
- Support the family to help them adjust, particularly if freedom from seizures leads to a more independent child.
- Support those children and families for whom surgery has been unsuccessful.

## Craniosynostosis

When massaging scars following hand surgery, the moisturizing cream should be one that does not contain vitamin E. This vitamin has been found to alter the healing process.

Sports can be undertaken once the surgeon has given the 'all-clear' following any surgery; however, head sports should always be avoided.

# Useful organizations

## Hydrocephalus

Association of Spina Bifida and Hydrocephalus (ASBAH), ASBAH House, 42 Park Rd, Peterborough PE1 2UQ. Telephone (01733) 555988. ASBAH provides advice and information through local networks regarding many issues concerning the care needs for those with hydrocephalus and spina bifida and their families. Information and publications are available on all aspects of care and management. Personal advice and support is provided wherever possible.

In Touch Trust, 10 Norman Road, Sale, Cheshire M33 3DF. Telephone (0161) 905 2440. Provides information and contacts for parents of children with special needs.

Network 81, 1–7 Woodfield Terrace, Stanstead, Essex CM24 8AJ. Telephone (01279) 647 414. Offers advice to parents of children with special educational needs.

National Association of Toy and Leisure Libraries, Play Matters, 68 Churchway, London NW1 1LT. Telephone (0207) 387 9592. Provides information on appropriate toys.

National Library for the Handicapped Child, Reach Resource Centre, Wellington House, Wellington Road, Wokingham, Berks RG40 2AG. Telephone (01734) 89101. Resource centre for children whose disabilities affect their reading, language and communication skills.

## Spinal abnormalities in children

Association of Spina Bifida and Hydrocephalus (ASBAH), ASBAH House, 42 Park Rd, Peterborough PE1 2UQ. Telephone (01733) 555988.

Association of Wheelchair Children, 33 Humerstone Road, London E13 9NL. Telephone (0208) 552 6561. Provides specialized teaching. Promotes independence and mobility.

Disability Alliance, Universal House, 88 Wenworth Street, London E1 7SA. Telephone (0207) 247 8776. Rights advice (0207) 247 8763.

Voluntary Council for Handicapped Children, National Children's Bureau, 8 Wakley Street, London EC1V 7QE. Telephone (0207) 843 6000. Provides information and 'signposting'.

Write Away, 29 Crawford Street, London W1H 1LP. Telephone (0207) 724 0878. Finds penfriends for children with special needs and their siblings.

## Brain tumours

Association for Children with Life-threatening or Terminal Conditions and their Families (ACT-NOW), 65 St Michael's Hill, Bristol BS2 8DZ. Telephone (0117) 922 1556.

BACUP, 3 Bath Place, Rivington Street, London EC2A JR. Telephone (0207) 613 2121. Trained nurses provide information and support to families, related to cancer.

British Association for Counselling, 1 Regent Place, Rugby, Warwickshire CV21 2PJ. Telephone (01788) 550899.

British Brain Tumour Association, 9 Roehampton Drive, Crosby, Merseyside L23 7XD. Telephone (0151) 929 3339.

Childhood Cancer Research Group, University of Oxford, 57 Woodstock Road, Oxford OX2 6HJ. Telephone (01865) 310030.

Child Bereavement Trust, Brindley House, 4 Burkes Road, Beaconsfield, Buckinghamshire. Telephone (01628) 488101.

Child Death Helpline. Telephone (0800) 282 986.

Hospice Information Service, St Christopher's Hospice, 51–59 Lawrie Park Road, London SE26 6DZ. Telephone (0208) 778 9252.

Macmillan Cancer Relief, Anchor House, 15–19 Britten Street, London SW3 3TZ. Telephone (0207) 351 7811.

National Association of Staff Support (NASS), 9 Caradon Close, Woking, Surrey GU21 3DU. Telephone (01483) 771599.

Rainbow Trust, Wyvern House, 1 Church Road, Great Bookham, Nr Leatherhead, Surrey KT23 3PD. Telephone (01372) 59055. Provides domicillary workers for terminally ill children.

Radiotherapy Action Group Exposure (Rage), 24 Lockett Gardens, Manchester M3 6BJ. Telephone (0161) 839 2927. Support and advice for those suffering radiation damage.

Royal College of Nursing Counselling Service, 9–11 Crown Hill, Croydon, Surrey CR0 1RZ. Telephone (01345) 697064.

Sargent Cancer Care for Children, 14 Abingdon Road, London W8 6AF. Telephone (0207) 565 5100.

UK Brain Tumour Resource Directory, 22 Cambridge Road, Aldershot, Hampshire GU11 3JZ. Telephone (01252) 653897.

United Kingdom Children's Cancer Study Group (UKCCSG), University of Leicester, Department of Epidemiology and Public Health, 22–28 Princess Road West, Leicester LE1 6TP. Telephone (0116) 252 3280.

# Epilepsy

Action for Sick Kids Trust, 10 Hill View Terrace, Ilminster, Somerset TA19 9AL. Helps severely disabled children to lead full and independent lives.

British Epilepsy Association, Anstey House, 40 Hanover Square, Leeds LS3 1BE. Helpline telephone (0800) 30 90 30. Resources available include *Epilepsy and the Child,* the *Parents and Young Children's Information Pack,* which contains a video and leaflets aimed at the child under 12, and the *Parents and Adolescents' Information Package,* which contains a video and leaflet aimed at teenagers and their parents.

The Family Fund, PO Box 50, York YO1 2ZX. Telephone (01904) 621115. Provides financial assistance for families caring for severely disabled children.

Voluntary Council for Handicapped Children, National Children's Bureau, 8 Wakley Street. London EC1V 7QE. Telephone (0207) 843 6000. Represents major agencies working with families of children with disabilities.

## Paediatric head injury

Children's Head Injury Trust, Radcliffe Infirmary, Woodstock Road, Oxford OX2 6HE. Telephone (01865) 224786.

Children's Trust, Tadworth Court, Tadworth KT20 5RU. Telephone (01737) 357171. Offers care, treatment and education to children with exceptional needs and profound disabilities, as well as short-term respite care.

Disabled Living Foundation, 380–384 Harrow Road, London W9 2HU. Telephone (0207) 289 6111.

Headway, 7 King Edward Court, King Edward Street, Nottingham NG1 1EW. Telephone (0115) 924 0800.

Independent Resource Centre. Special Needs, 112 Grove Park, Knutsford, Cheshire WA16 8QD. Telephone (01565) 632666. Provides a national helpline special education service for parents of children with disabilities aged 0–19 years.

Network 81, 1–7 Woodfield Terrace, Stansted, Essex CM24 8AJ. Telephone (01279) 647415. Advice with regard to educational needs.

REMAP, Hazeldene, Igtham, Sevenoaks, Kent TN15 9AD. Telephone (01732) 883818. Technical help for disabled children.

Whizz-Kidds, 215 Vauxhall Bridge Road, London SW1V 1EN. Telephone (0207) 233 6600. Mobility aids provider for disabled children.

Brain Injury Rehabilitation Trust, 32 Market Place, Burgess Hill, West Sussex RH15 9NP. Telephone (01908) 640775.

Brain and Spine Foundation, 7 Winchester Place, Kennington Park, Cranner Road, London SW9 6EJ. Telephone (0800) 8081000 – freephone for advice from nurses.

## Craniosynostosis

Craniofacial support group, 44 Helmsdale Road, Leamington Spa, Warwickshire CV32 7DW. Telephone (01926) 334629. This supplies a network of families with craniofacial conditions such as Apert's and Crouzon's syndromes. It provides the following leaflets: *The Genetic Background to Craniosynostosis; Craniosynostosis; Apert's Syndrome; Crouzon's Syndrome; Hand Surgery; Pfeiffer/Clover Leaf Syndrome; Parental Aspects of Craniofacial Conditions; Saethre-Chotzen Syndrome; Your Child In Hospital; Glossary of Terms Associated with Craniosynostosis; Coping with Facial Disfigurement.*

Changing Faces, 1 and 2 Junction Mews, Paddington, London N1 9BN. Telephone (0207) 706 4232. Provides information and advice, social skills workshops and counselling, for anyone around Britain with a facial disfigurement, whatever the cause.

Let's Face It, 14 Fallowfield, Yateley, Surrey GU17 7LU. Telephone (01252) 879630. Provides a support network around the UK and other countries for those with facial disfigurements, particularly after cancer treatment.

# Index